For Enrique Mendez Jr., M.D.
Assistant Secretary of Defense for Health Affairs
with warmest regards

John C. Duff, M.D.
August 30, 1990

Health and Medical Aspects of Disaster Preparedness

NATO • Challenges of Modern Society

A series of edited volumes comprising multifaceted studies of contemporary problems facing our society, assembled in cooperation with NATO Committee on the Challenges of Modern Society.

Volume 1 AIR POLLUTION MODELING AND ITS APPLICATION I
Edited by C. De Wispelaere

Volume 2 AIR POLLUTION: Assessment Methodology and Modeling
Edited by Erich Weber

Volume 3 AIR POLLUTION MODELING AND ITS APPLICATION II
Edited by C. De Wispelaere

Volume 4 HAZARDOUS WASTE DISPOSAL
Edited by John P. Lehman

Volume 5 AIR POLLUTION MODELING AND ITS APPLICATION III
Edited by C. De Wispelaere

Volume 6 REMOTE SENSING FOR THE CONTROL OF MARINE POLLUTION
Edited by Jean-Marie Massin

Volume 7 AIR POLLUTION MODELING AND ITS APPLICATION IV
Edited by C. De Wispelaere

Volume 8 CONTAMINATED LAND: Reclamation and Treatment
Edited by Michael A. Smith

Volume 9 INTERREGIONAL AIR POLLUTION MODELING: The State of the Art
Edited by S. Zwerver and J. van Ham

Volume 10 AIR POLLUTION MODELING AND ITS APPLICATION V
Edited by C. De Wispelaere, Francis A. Schiermeier, and Noor V. Gillani

Volume 11 AIR POLLUTION MODELING AND ITS APPLICATION VI
Edited by Han van Dop

Volume 12 RISK MANAGEMENT OF CHEMICALS IN THE ENVIRONMENT
Edited by Hans M. Seip and Anders B. Heiberg

Volume 13 AIR POLLUTION MODELING AND ITS APPLICATION VII
Edited by Han van Dop

Volume 14 HEALTH AND MEDICAL ASPECTS OF DISASTER PREPAREDNESS
Edited by John C. Duffy

Health and Medical Aspects of Disaster Preparedness

Edited by
John C. Duffy
Assistant Surgeon General
Gillis W. Long Hansen's Disease Center
Carville, Louisiana

Published in cooperation with
NATO Committee on the Challenges of Modern Society
PLENUM PRESS • NEW YORK AND LONDON

Library of Congress Cataloging in Publication Data

Health and medical aspects of disaster preparedness / edited by John C. Duffy.
p. cm.—(NATO challenges of modern society; v. 14)
"Published in cooperation with NATO Committee on the Challenges of Modern Society."
"Report of a four-year pilot study on health and medical aspects of disaster preparedness, held between 1985 and 1989 in Washington, D.C."—T.p. verso.
Includes bibliographical references.
ISBN 0-306-43495-4
1. Disaster relief—Congresses. 2. Disaster medicine—Congresses. 3. Emergency medical services—Congresses. I. Duffy, John C. (John Charles), 1934- . II. North Atlantic Treaty Organization. Committee on the Challenges of Modern Society. III. Series.
[DNLM: 1. Disaster Planning. 2. Emergencies. 3. Emergency Medical Services. 4. Public Health. WB 105 H434 1989]
RA645.9.H43 1990
362.1'8—dc20
DNLM/DLC 90-6789
for Library of Congress CIP

Proceedings of a four-year pilot study on
Health and Medical Aspects of Disaster Preparedness,
held in Washington, D.C.

A Division of Plenum Publishing Corporation
233 Spring Street, New York, N.Y. 10013

Printed in the United States of America

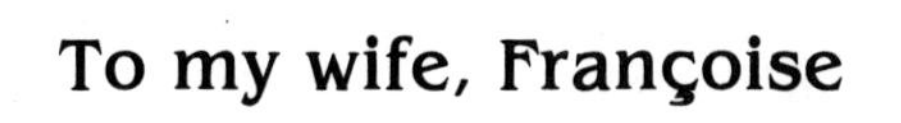
To my wife, Françoise

PREFACE

The study of Health and Medical Aspects of Disaster Preparedness was approved by NATO/CCMS in 1985 with the first pilot study meeting in June of that year. The pilot study, under the leadership of the United States and Belgium, focused on the current status of disaster preparedness in participating nations. An objective look was taken at the availability or resources to cope with disasters from an international standpoint. The types of disaster settings that were reviewed in the study included the following:

(1) Earthquakes, floods, hurricanes, avalanches

(2) Nuclear power plant accidents or spills

(3) Water and aircraft accidents

(4) Building fires, building collapses

(5) Contamination by hazardous chemicals or biological waste

(6) Civil disturbances

A disaster can strike anywhere at any time. Some nations and local communities have well-developed disaster plans with which to meet catastrophic situations. The fact is that most communities are without written and coordinated disaster plans which offer their citizens the most effective and comprehensive protection in these unexpected and often critical situations.

Disaster has been defined as a sudden event which involves large numbers of people and results in loss of life, serious injury and property loss, together with a severe disruption of community organization and services. In the United States, thousands of people are killed and injured in disasters every year. Thus, disasters constitute a serious problem in both individual and public health terms in this country alone.

Disasters can be classified as natural and man-made. Natural disasters include earthquakes, floods, tsunamis, hurricanes, avalanches, epidemics, droughts, and famines. Those which are considered man-made include explosions, fires, civil riots and disturbances, major transportation accidents, chemical and radiological pollution. Clearly, the industrialization which has occurred in so many countries throughout the world contributes to many disasters and potential disasters.

In many areas of the world, natural events produce a constant threat of disaster such as in earthquake, flood, hurricane and avalanche prone areas. One would expect that in these areas, fairly well developed and coordinated disaster plans would exist that could cope with these events, should they occur. However, the problem with disaster preparedness plans is that preparedness requires that plans be prepared, coordinated, tested or exercised, and updated in order to be ready for any event, including those which may never occur. Unless a national disaster strategy is designed to accommodate and coordinate existing organizations which may have other primary missions, the cost of preparedness becomes prohibitive. The organizational aspects of disaster planning emerge as areas of prime importance. It becomes necessary to engage all relevant existing organizations in disaster planning efforts with the assignment of clear role designations and clear lines of authority, along with the declaration of lead agencies.

Increased industrialization and technological advances have brought nations closer together. Interdependency and sociologic ties make it expedient for emergency planning to account for the potential assistance which nations might provide to one another in connection with potential and actual mass disasters. This dictates the need for a national plan which accommodates international activities.

The many organizations and people involved in providing assistance to victims of a disaster must be cognizant of the fundamental principles involved in disaster management. These include preventing the occurrence of the disaster; prevention of occurrence of additional casualties after the initial impact; rescue of individuals; provision of emergency care to the injured; evacuation of the injured to appropriate medical installations or aid stations; the provision of definitive medical care for the seriously ill and injured; relocation of residents of the disaster area; and the promotion of the reconstruction of the disaster area and lives of the victims.

Successful disaster planning must impact on several factors which are relevant to operations in disaster settings. Good communications (management and medical) are essential to successful disaster rescue operations. Triage, the classifying and prioritizing of casualties in order that each victim is assured the medical attention which is required, will be facilitated by a standardized tagging or sorting system. Categorization of hospital facilities assures that victims are transported to facilities which are capable of providing medical care as required. Immediate and coordinated transportation is imperative for those victims who have life-threatening injuries and require institutional emergency medical care. Also, these procedures will be required for many of the victims with injuries which may not be as serious. Adequate disaster planning includes arrangements for needed manpower, such as professional medical and nursing personnel, paraprofessionals, and volunteers who have the knowledge and skills required to provide care for victims of a disaster. These interrelated and interdependent activities require an organization for management of all resources at the disposal of a community if its residents are to have the most effective system available for coping with disasters. Local, state, regional, national and international cooperation will assure that most individuals in stricken countries receive the care and services needed in these emergency situations.

Both member and non-member nations have sent representatives to pilot study meetings over the three year history of this study. Among the most frequent countries who contributed to the pilot study were:

Canada
United Kingdom

Italy
Greece
Germany
Portugal
France
Netherlands
Spain
Kuwait

In addition, there have been representatives from the Pan American Health Organization.

Two pilot study meetings were exceptionally valuable in terms of their contribution to the final report. In July 1986, pilot study members participated in the first full scale national disaster exercise in the United States. The second meeting, hosted by the Belgians in the spring of 1987, was in Antwerp. There the participants toured major industrial plants and installations and reviewed their disaster response plans.

It is clear that disaster planning at the national level is sparse and almost non-existent between contiguous nations. This publication looks at examples of disaster plans; hypothetical models for investigation of health and medical aspects of disaster preparedness; data collection; the role of stress in the disaster scenario; joint civil/military contributions, among the more important topics.

One of the very important contributions of NATO/CCMS is the support provided by their Fellowships program. Three contributors to this book were supported by Fellowship grants: Doctors Lund, Baxter, and Antonini.

The exceptional effort required to communicate with authors, organize and prepare manuscripts for publication was carried out by my secretary, Laurie Bourgeois. Without her dedication and commitment, this book could not have been finished.

Appreciation must also be given to all the participants who shared their expertise with us. We are particularly grateful to Alan Sielen, United States Coordinator for NATO/CCMS Activities, and NATO/CCMS for providing the mechanism and support for the study.

Finally, a special thank you to the Belgians who, as co-leaders of this pilot study, have given generously of their time and resources. In this regard, special mention must be given to Daniel Van Daele, Director General, and Etienne L. Pelfrene, Ministry of Public Health and The Family, Brussels, Belgium

John C. Duffy, M.D., FAPA, FAsMA
Assistant Surgeon General
U.S. Public Health Service

CONTENTS

DISASTER MEDICINE - AN OVERALL RESPONSE TO DISASTER SITUATIONS

NATO-Joint Civil/Military Group Report
Brussels, Belgium

THE PROBLEM - DISASTERS

1. Definition

Our first objective should be to determine exactly "what is a disaster." A good number of definitions have been developed by researchers on the matter; however, some essential medical aspects seem to have been forgotten.

WHO defines DISASTER as an "act of nature or of man which may mean a menace serious or great enough to justify emergency aid, in which extensive material damage is followed by tragic losses of human life and large numbers of victims whose injuries are invariably serious." However, if there are instances where the devastation is so massive that there is no question about the meaning of the word, more limited disaster situations resulting in mass casualties require an exact definition, in order to allow proper medical action.

In all these unexpected events, the immediate emergency medical needs of the ill or injured are among the highest priorities. To achieve the most effective medical response is one of the major issues, because each hospital, each system, each region has its own limit of response capabilities concerning manpower, equipment, organization and training. On the other hand, some regions don't ever possess an acceptable system, and require help from other areas or countries - so called "mutual aid."

(a) First let us imagine a system that was conceived to respond to broader situations than just day-to-day operations according to the needs of a community at a certain time. However, when unexpected outbreaks of illness or injuries occur, other levels of operations should be considered.

- Multiple casualty situations that temporarily may stress the system's availability of resources, and may have little impact on the response capability of the total existing Emergency Medical Services (EMS);

- Mass casualty situations that clearly exceed the response capabilities of the system and stress the emergency capabilities of multiple hospital facilities, rendering EMS unable to respond to any other incidents for several hours;

Health and Medical Aspects of Disaster Preparedness
Edited by J.C. Duffy
Plenum Press, New York, 1990

- Full disaster situations render all capabilities of EMS completely exhausted. The number, location and accessibility of casualties overwhelm even the best organized and equipped emergency medical system.

- The mobility of the field EMS may be lost and the hospital may have suffered damage so that they are unable to use their full resources, and national or international help is needed.

(b) Secondly, let us imagine a small disaster or just the outbreak of multiple casualties in rural areas where health resources are limited or non-existent. In medical terms such incidents should be considered very near to full disaster.

In summary: each one of these situations may be a disaster if the medical response is insufficient.

But physical injuries are not the only medical aspect of a disaster. All catastrophes have, in several degrees, psychological effects on survivors, whose reactions usually occur in three phases: impact, reactive emotional disturbances, and the survivor syndrome.

Public health problems, like environmental sanitation and epidemic diseases frequently arise together with the disaster and according to its extent. However, the severity of such health problems often does not correspond to the impact they have on public opinion.

2. TYPES OF DISASTER

Generally, the classification of disasters gives a rough indication of the probable number of casualties, type of injuries and duration of the event. However, the great variety of disasters from country to country and the differences in emergency medical services available, render agreement on classification of difficult issue.

In a disaster situation various parameters should be identified: SIZE, LOCATION, AREA, EVACUATION OF SITE AND CAUSE. This fact underlines the need of an effort for a uniform notification which will allow at the same time a standard classification of disasters, both nationally and internationally.

Disasters fall into the first level division of natural and man-made. Those include earthquakes, cyclones, hurricanes and floods. Among the man-induced are emergencies resulting from technological breakdowns, airplane crashes and roadway accidents, sea disasters, fire or explosion (including bombing), large scale poisoning, evil unrest, terrorism, and war.

Another classification, no doubt relevant for planning, divides disaster into two groups according to the fact of physical or organizational structures and human resources of the EMS having been damaged or not.

Nevertheless, each hospital should have its own classification of disasters in order to allow a phased response: limited, general or distant, based on the number of casualties they have the capability to treat and on the location of event.

THE MEDICAL RESPONSE

In a disaster situation resulting in mass casualties, the medical response is certainly the most important component within the global reaction of the community.

Although a relationship between EMS and other agencies involved in emergency activities (civil defense, fire, police, military) is obviously necessary, in many countries it doesn't exist formally. Since they must work together on a stress-filled scenario they should carry out joint planning and training activities. Such a task becomes easier when the establishment of an integrated EMS System is under way.

DISASTER MEDICINE

Returning to what has been stated before concerning the problem of disasters, it becomes easy to understand the meaning of disaster medicine.

The main role of EMS is in the field of the immediate response - the first line of defense is the treatment of casualties - represents the most relevant part of the medical response that also includes other aspects linked to preventive medicine.

Articles, editorials and books identify DISASTER MEDICINE as a "sudden concentration of casualties that overwhelms the existing medical facilities."

The medical definition of Disaster as "an unexpected and excessive request for emergency medical care that exhausts the available resources," not only renders the quantitative parameter of the definition as evident, but also lets us understand the qualitative components and the level of response required.

In those cases in which it is impossible to maintain the delivery of an acceptable standard of care to a small number of major surgical casualties all arriving at the same time, it may be justified to declare a state of disaster. When, on the contrary, the arrivals are well spaced, such cases may probably be treated through regular facilities. This means that each hospital and each region should develop some guidelines for the definition of a disaster situation according to its ability to cope, or in other words, according to its DISRUPTION RATIO. Such guidelines should also include who has the authority and the responsibility to declare a disaster.

In summary: Disaster Medicine should be considered as a discipline linked to an expansion of clinical practice of Emergency (The optimization of the resources and immediate response components: Triage, immediate care, casualty evacuation, communications, psychological assistance in community), and to some aspects of Preventive Medicine (prevention of disasters and response planning). A phased response disaster plan will allow a flexible and progressive mobilization of health resources according to the type and extent of the event.

A. COMPONENTS OF IMMEDIATE RESPONSE SYSTEM

1. TRIAGE

Triage is a French-rooted word which has been used to describe the initial sorting out of war victims. In a mass casualty, the critically injured will be given immediate life support and should be first priority in treatment. Less injured patients or dying patients with no hope of survival should be handled later.

Following the natural process of treatment of the injured in a mass casualty, dynamic procedures of triage should be performed not only at the scene, but also at the entrance to the hospital and in the hospital.

(a) At the Scene of the Incident

At the scene of the incident the first task should be a quick assessment of the extent of the medical problem, with a view to the development of the most adequate response plan. A secure staging area for the reception and triage of patients should be identified, eventually supported by a Field Command Post Unit, with the capability of communicating via radio with the EOC (Emergency Operations Center), with the hospitals and the ambulances, according to the plans previously written. All the patients should proceed through triage staging area, to prevent confusion at the Hospital admission services.

The next step should be the establishment of treatment priorities and evacuation and the completion of individual identification tags which should be attached to the patient until his admission at the hospital. In these tags the rescuers should record details concerning first assessment and treatment.

The main problem for a medical team operating in disaster situations is the definition of priorities. This is a difficult task which requires expertise and psychological balance, and which should only be assigned to a senior doctor preferably consultant in emergency medicine or trauma surgeon. Triage must be based not only on knowledge about pathology, pathophysiology, prognosis or injuries but also on combined injuries in correlation to severity or time factor and on available capabilities. The limiting circumstances of triage should by no means forget the ethical principle of "duty of guard" for every human life.

Emergency treatment should be performed by the other members of the team: junior physicians, nurses and paramedics, but never by the senior doctor whose responsibility is accurate and appropriate triage.

Since the number of patients exceeds the available resources, it is necessary to select those patients who will be able to survive and eventually be treated in hospital facilities and those who will inevitably die.

Deaths should be dully confirmed by physicians who are to record the fact on the individual identification tag, in order to prevent duplication of services.

When triage at the scene and evacuation of the survivors has been accomplished, it is important that appropriate teams perform the management of the dead, identifying and removing the corpses, so as to avoid decomposition at the scene.

(b) Triage at the Entrance of the Hospital

Patient's admission to Emergency Department should be effected through one entrance only, as to prevent the slightly injured patients from obtaining immediate treatment, thus hampering the urgent management of the really critically injured.

Triage upon arrival is no doubt the most important under a technical point of view; it is the key for an effective management of sudden arrival of a large number of casualties. It should be run by a senior experience physician. Resuscitation and follow-up treatment should be performed by other physicians on duty.

The triage area should be wide and located at the ED entrance. Immediately adjacent there should be conceived and equipped in such a way that it will allow the optimization of its functions in disaster situations. If necessary, the waiting room should be adapted for this purpose.

(c) In Hospital Triage

The arrival of a large number of victims at the ED will result in patient overload, mainly in the surgery and X-Ray departments. All patients with surgical indication should be placed in the same room as to allow the senior surgeon in charge to definitively evaluate the priorities while the other surgeons of the team operate in the theatre. The minor surgery area also requires the presence of a senior surgeon to prevent the possibility that the seriously injured patients be brought inadvertently, and also to make the decision of when wounds should be closed or left open for delayed primary suture.

The necessity to obtain vacant beds in wards requires that triage should still be performed by a senior surgeon who will also sort out patients for discharge.

Radiological investigation should be limited to emergencies. Triage at the X-Ray Department is unique due to the fact that patients are brought in after resuscitation has been initiated. The examination requests may come from different areas and priorities should be identified in a very accurate and sensible way by a senior Radiologist who is to select only the most urgent. The other requests should be delayed for a later and more calm occasion.

Evaluation of Priorities

In general terms, victims could be classified in three large groups, according to the severity of the injuries and consequent evaluation of priorities for treatment and evacuation.

GROUP 1 - Includes patients who need immediate care to survive:

- Serious respiratory distress;
- Massive bleeding;
- Trauma amputation of the limbs, or serious fracture with bleeding;
- Cardiac wounds;
- Shock; serious burns;
- Head; trauma; unconsciousness;

GROUP 2 - Patients who require urgent treatment within 6 hours:

- Pre-shock;
- Serious fractures with no bleeding;
  simple fracture of the femur;
  Abdominal contusions;
- Head trauma without focal signs;

GROUP 3 - Patients who do not require urgent treatment. Treatment may be deferred.

There is still a 4th Group, strategically associated with Group 3 which comprises those patients who are so badly injured that no treatment will save their lives.

In the above list only the most common examples are listed. The triage officer should be prepared for an accurate evaluation of each situation including associate injuries.

In triage, a uniform system of patient tagging should be defined, either letters A, B, C, numbers 1, 2, 3, colors Red, Yellow, Green or still easily understandable animal drawings like bird, hare or turtle in order to express the relative emergency degree in immediate care and the priority of evacuation.

In summary: We could state the Triage should be a continual procedure while there are victims to be treated. It is easy to understand that the clinical evolution of a given patient may change at any time, therefore requiring a re-classification in a short period of time.

Specific Aspects in Triage

In Triage some specific aspects should be considered:

Childhood - Children have peculiar problems in diagnosis and emergency care. Their presence among disaster victims (10% of the population are children in Europe) may justify the need for a pediatrician in Triage areas.

The degree of life-threatening injuries in children, their need for care, their living patterns, and their social environment, are clearly different from those of adults.

Brain Injuries - Triage can be based upon the Glasgow coma scale. However, the existence of combined injuries leading to hypotension and hypoxia should be considered before allotting the victim to a triage category. Any victim with evidence of head trauma, but with minimal signs of brain failure should be given a special triage category in order to timely identify the first signs of neurological deterioration.

Burns - Burn situations with multiple victims follow the general principle of Triage, but some modifications in the usual priority system should be established.

The usual method of ascertaining the overall severity of the injury, the percentage of body surface burn, is insufficient. Each patients should be evaluated according to the depth of burn, the area of the body involved, and the ambulatory state.

In mass casualty situations the patient with 2nd and 3rd degree burns involving more than 40% of the body surface would probably not survive. He should only receive definitive treatment after all patients in higher priority groups have received adequate therapy.

The major effort should be directed towards administering treatment to those having 15% - 40% body surface area burns, and to those who have less than 15% but still require special care.

Chemicals - Release and escape of industrial chemicals into the environment (water, air, sea) may cause epidemics of massive intoxications. Acute poisoning with organic-phosphates shows clearly the need for particular care.

Chemicals (continued)

The toxicity of the hazardous materials must be assessed before triage in order to avoid that rescuers become casualties themselves. Field decontamination of the "hot area" has priority and a "clean zone" should be established where triage and immediate care should be carried out.

A data bank on toxins should be easily accessible, not only for planning rescuing in high risk areas but also for the management of casualties.

Nuclear Accidents - In general, emergency professionals are not training in the medical aspects of radiation injury and are dramatically uninformed about a limited radiation hazard: industrial or laboratory accidents, nuclear weapons tests or reactor malfunctions.

Psychological stress of the victim is communicated to the emergency workers troubling their capability of handling the patients who are often physically injured. EMS personnel should at least be informed of the fact that the irradiated patient is not a danger for the attendants. On the other hand, the contaminated patient is not a medical emergency but does need to be handled with special and quite simple precautions.

2. IMMEDIATE CARE

In Disaster Medicine, the concept of the "golden hour" in the prognosis of the multiple trauma patient remains critical. However, actions like immediate care and stabilization of the victim prior to transportation, which are emphasized in emergency medicine, are regarded in a different perspective.

Resuscitology, through the scientific survey of acute situations which lead to death (life-threatening injuries, terminal status, clinical death) and their reversability (emergency and long-term resuscitation), has allowed significant improvement in resuscitation skills, operative-care room and intensive life-support of multiple injured victims.

On the other hand, the forensic methodologies for studying autopsy records and terminal hospital records may contribute to the knowledge of the various patterns of injury and their incidence. This fact allied to the performance of adequate rescue and resuscitation techniques will certainly reduce the number of fatalities.

Research demands a critical re-evaluation of rescue techniques and shows clearly the importance of prompt life-support and rapidly available intensive hospital care.

In disaster situations the disproportion between the needs and the available resources begins at the scene of the event. Therefore, only essential first aid should be delivered on site in order not to delay evacuation and consequently in-hospital initial definitive treatment. If, by any chance, the evacuation becomes difficult, the possibility of getting more advance life-support should be available.

Planning for immediate care at the scene should be simple, so as to allow an easy adjustment to the unexpected situation. Treatment procedures should be very similar to daily emergency care, in order to obtain a prompt and effective response.

RESPONSE PATTERNS IN IMMEDIATE CARE

First Aid

Such training in immediate care should be considered as complimentary of general education, in order to meet the necessities of everyday life. It should start in childhood at primary school and continue until adolescence and high school.

Having in mind that many disasters may occur in isolated areas, and considering that a few minutes may decide upon survival of many victims, training in first aid procedures should be implemented constantly.

For this purpose a basic disaster kit designed to provide minimal but adequate resuscitation at the scene should be available.

Primary Health Care

Primary health care personnel should be motivated and trained to perform such activities. In the immediate aftermath of a disaster, this personnel should be responsible for information data collection, as well as for quick and simple reports of the situation in what concerns damages, operating resources and expected needs.

Procedures should be developed for the rapid transmission of the data to the decision makers for their evaluation, their circulation and their feedback. Since no system of information can be improvised, this reporting system should be integrated into a national health information system and activated in case of disaster.

The tasks of health care personnel should be clearly defined and should include, among others: assess and report of the situation, provision of rescue and first aid services, and implementation of community participation. They should also have the capability of checking supplies and providing for coordination of sanitary, veterinary and community services.

Primary health care personnel should join their efforts according to a pre-determined plan. Their first responsibility should be to perform triage, sorting out the dead and the injured, and provide health care to survivors. This personnel should be trained in life-saving procedures as clearing of airways, controlling of bleeding and treatment of shock and cardiac arrest.

The medical intervention in difficult fields demands adjusted dress and survival equipment for the medical team. A transportable kit containing equipment for triage and immediate resuscitation is also necessary.

Emergency Care

The provision of emergency care involves the establishment of medical and surgical treatment to the injured at the scene. Emergency care should be performed by well-trained personnel, who should start to act as soon as possible after the disaster has struck. Emergency care may be started at the scene, during transportation (ambulance, helicopter or other means), or at the hospital Emergency Department.

Once Hospitals and Health Centers have been notified, they should activate their contingency plans and mobilize their resources to the scene. They may deliver medical or rescue teams, trained in life-saving procedures, depending on the extent of the disaster.

In the field of immediate care delivery, we should consider basically two models, which may function as complementary phases of treatment.

(a) Mobile Intensive Care Units

Very similar to ambulance vehicles operating in the pre-hospital phase of the EMS system. The crews know the region very well and their interventions are very often related to rescue problems. They should be staffed by one physician or nurse, proficient in life-support skills and should have the capability of arriving at the scene as soon as possible. Crews should not only be well trained in routine primary life-support but also have the ability of performing advanced life-support procedures.

Considering that in mass casualties the only possible treatment at the scene is to institute life-saving procedures (airway, bleeding, shock) the necessary equipment should be available. The unit consists of a modified ambulance containing resuscitation equipment, an intravenous kit, a dressing kit, fracture equipment, burn kits, a doctor bag, a minor injury box, communication equipment and safety equipment.

At the scene all the units report to the Field Command Post and act according to the Triage performed by the senior physician in charge.

This type of unit results in the optimization of the EMS pre-hospital ambulance vehicle enforced by the presence of an expert physician or nurse from the ED, according to the previous plan, or may be instituted independent from the system, manned by surplus ED personnel, with a view to enhancing the activities of the first or acting in the most needful areas.

(b) The Mobile Hospital

The model is particularly suggested in cases when the disaster has taken place far from hospital facilities, or when these have also been struck.

The Mobile Hospital is also suggested in cases when the number of victims exceeds the capabilities of the available medical resources.

The model consists of a sophisticated Mobile Intensive Care and Surgical Unit, containing an emergency room, operating theatre, recovery room and one or more tented wards. It is fully equipped and is staffed by the necessary medical, nursing and auxiliary personnel. Sufficient stocks of drugs, emergency equipment, medical and surgical equipment should be available. Stocks of food for the staff should also be ready, so as to avoid utilization of the limited resources of the affected community.

The whole organization of this pattern requires that the function of each sector be defined and the equipment and the drugs be standardized.

The unit must be ready to respond very fast and may be set in the surroundings of the affected area. It should have the capability of providing advanced treatment to the severely injured victims who need surgical therapy, resuscitation, intensive care, preparing them for secondary transportation. It should also be able to provide treatment to light ambulatory cases.

The concept of this unit should be totally independent from any local system.

A plan for the relief of teams and the renewal of supplies should always be considered.

The coordination of the Mobile Hospital performance should be assigned to a local unified control, which should deploy the Unit and control its cooperations according to a predetermined National Disaster Plan.

3. CASUALTY EVACUATION AND TRANSPORTATION

In disaster situations several factors may influence the casualties evacuation. Among them we should consider not only the severity of the injury and the number of casualties but the terrain and the distance, the time factor, the refugee problem, etc.

These factors will certainly determine the most adequate type of transport, as well as the coordination of the available resources and the level of help required.

Generally, the majority of patients in a mass casualty will be multiple trauma victims. At the scene it is impossible to locate and stabilize each broken bone for every patient. As mentioned before, the most important is to sort out the casualties and treat the life-threatening systemic problems only.

In general terms, after triage and essential first aid procedures, patients should be duly packaged for transport very quickly. Continuity of care during evacuation should be assured by personnel trained in advanced life support. At the hospital, the victims will receive appropriate definitive treatment. In disaster situations it should be emphasized that only extremely urgent surgery should be performed outside the hospital.

The priorities for evacuation are assessed in the triage area that is also the loading site for ambulance and other transport. Radio communications will allow constantly assessment and coordination of the available resources.

The triage officer should know which facilities are available not only at his own hospital but also at neighboring hospitals, including the number and location of vacant beds, specialists and other medical staff on duty, operating theatres (the categorization of the involved hospitals in the medical response to disaster). This is a very important point for a correct distribution of the patients; some group 2 or group 3 victims may be sent to more distant hospitals so as not to overwhelm the nearest hospital.

General and specific safety rules of people evacuation should be disseminated by civil defense agencies.

Transportation capabilities require not only the optimization of the EMS system ambulances but also the cooperation of those of the military and volunteer agencies.

Different types of vehicles may be used in disaster situation. We will just refer the most important means of transportation of critical patients.

Ambulances conceived for this purpose have a day-to-day emergency routine but more duties than just the transportation of supine patients. In general, the patient compartment can accommodate two rescuers and two litter patients so positioned that at least one of them can receive intensive lifesaving care during transit. Such a vehicle should have equipment and supplies for the delivery of emergency care at the scene and during transportation, and must have a two-way radio communication capability between the ambulance and the EOC (Emergency Operations Center) dispatcher and between the ambulance and the hospital.

Equipment should be standardized for basic and advanced life-support as to allow an easy adaptation to any type of vehicle according to the victim's needs and the health personnel capabilities.

The value of the helicopter as a means of evacuation is nowadays recognized. After having been wounded or injured, the most critical period of time will occur within the first few hours after the incident. Therefore, quick evacuation reduces shock and infection at least 60%. In this aspect, the helicopter can play a vital role, but should only be used to evacuate individuals with injuries or illnesses threatening life, limb or sight; in such instances delay in treatment may result in death or permanent disability.

The capabilities and the liability of helicopter evacuation must be known and considered. Its successful utilization in war has resulted in a greater utilization by the military, which should be "translated" into comparable civilian emergency programs.

Another aspect that should be considered is the ambulatory and also the so called "horizontal taxi work", usually performed by volunteer fire brigades. Their co-operation in mass casualties is most valuable; they should be co-ordinated and supervised by the same authority.

Finally, the need for a global and integrated transportation should be taken into consideration. In a disaster, it may be most effective to place all collective vehicles, such as buses or trucks, and accessible fuel stocks under a central authority. To transport health and supervisory personnel, to carry supplies and equipment, to evacuate the victims, to remove the bodies, are tasks that should be under the co-ordination of the same central authority.

4. COMMUNICATIONS

Communications setup is an essential component of any EMS system. Ideally, the national health services network should have communication equipment permanently available. This is important not only in day-today emergency operations but also for the execution of disaster plans.

In these situations, the resources of the EMS are often insufficient to cover control and co-ordination of the agencies involved. Telephone and teleprinter services as well as Citizen Band (CB) play important roles in disasters mainly in the alert phase. Radio communications within the EMS should be implemented, as they allow health facilities and relief personnel in the field to communicate. The possibility of using satellite transmissions should be considered in the event of a catastrophe.

5. PSYCHOLOGICAL ASSISTANCE

Disasters change the lives of the people involved, sometimes seriously, sometimes permanently. The world which has been safe and calm suddenly becomes a strange and terrifying place of uncertainty and unpredictability. The man's ability to adapt is insufficient and people react under emotional crisis without being mentally ill.

Psychological reactions in disasters are classically described in three phases: Impact phase, reactive emotional disturbances and the survivor's syndrome. It is important to have in mind that these effects may strike three different groups: The responders (doctors, firemen, police, etc), the survivors and the relatives.

Psychological assistance for responders in coping with the stress of a disaster should begin before the event occurs, through training sessions.

Assistance for survivors in the community should be provided by mental health professionals or members of the clergy visiting the family of the victim, in order that the behavior of these people may temporarily change as they adjust to their new circumstances.

Some specific services, like baby-sitting, cooking, financial support, may be needed in the phase of disruption. The victims and their families should be encouraged to make use of them.

Disaster response plans should take into account these very real needs.

6. HOSPITAL

The hospital is the fundamental piece of medical response to a disaster through its emergency department and the pre-hospital care system.

First priority in the community response is to know the categorization of its hospital. Each region, each country should have a well-established network of hospital categorization. The implementation of Emergency Medical Services Systems with the aim of getting a high level of care in day-to-day emergency operations is the key of having a good medical response. The practice of a good emergency care routine is the best way to get training for disaster situation response. We shouldn't forget that in unexpected and troubling situations of catastrophe, personnel have the natural tendency to work according to the routine patterns. The therapeutic protocols should be simple and flexible so that their implementation and adaptation may be easy and quick.

The definition of a disaster in medical terms has been mentioned before. Each hospital and each system should have established their own disruption plan, according to their capabilities. They should have an elaborate plan for a phased response in case a catastrophe occurs.

B. PREVENTION AND PLANNING

1. GENERAL POINTS OF CONSIDERATION

It has been said that the scientific basis for approaching Disaster Medicine may be set through Preventive Medicine techniques of investigation. The use of an epidemiological model clearly shows the necessity for pre-planning disaster situations.

In fact, disaster situations resulting in mass casualties should be regarded as sudden epidemics. Therefore, collecting and processing of data regarding the incidence of injuries and illness, made as early as possible, and according to geographic and demographic basis, will help establish the timely response for the location and treatment of victims. The same procedures are useful for the prevention of further occurrence of illness and injuries.

A true mass casualty incident doesn't occur frequently, perhaps only once in the career of most emergency medical personnel. Therefore, being a comparative rarity, to gain the necessary skills and expertise to manage disaster, the only possibility the personnel have is through training and performance according to a pre-event planning.

The survey of the causes and characteristics of disasters occurred in the past helps investigation procedures as well as the evaluation of the difficulties at the scene, and provides the guidelines for planning the medical response.

Disasters take many forms. Natural disasters, like earthquakes, floods, hurricanes, involve a variable area and bring frequently the problem of breakdown in communications, roads and supplies of electricity and water. Man-made disasters are usually due to fires, explosions, bombing, structural collapses, train or plane crashes; generally they are not involved with major disruption of transportation.

The risk of a disaster may be predicted to a certain degree and in certain circumstances. Disasters may be avoided or reduced to a minimum by the proper use of available technological resources, supported by an efficient organization.

(a) Few health care systems have undertaken realistic overall planning for handling large numbers of casualties;

(b) In those cases in which medical problems have different degrees of severity the response time may not be the most important issue, but the overall coordination of the response between field forces and the hospitals is always relevant;

(c) Accurate on-site assessment of the needs for emergency medical care almost never occurs, the reason for this fact being the atmosphere of uncertainty and distress in the first hours following a disaster consistent with the absence of trained personnel;

Such facts lead almost always to a disproportionate relation between the needs, the aid and materials delivered to the site;

(d) Meaningful on-site Triage is seldom possible in disasters, due to several factors: small number of emergency medical personnel, overcrowded emergency facilities, treatment of the less seriously injured just as the critical patients begin arriving, etc;

(e) Poor intra and inter-organizational communications are common in disasters due to equipment failure, absence of trained personnel, distorted messages or other reasons;

(f) The removal, transportation and distribution of casualties in disasters leave much to be desired, partly due to the tendency for the victims to be found by non-medically trained persons who do not understand Triage, use private vehicles or choose the nearest hospital disregarding its capabilities;

(g) There is a generalized tendency in all emergency medical systems to pay little or no attention to accurate record keeping in disaster situations.

Generally, three major issues, administrative rather than clinical, are a constant in all disaster operations:

(i) Command and Control
(ii) Coordination
(iii) Communications

The need for a realistic overall planning and an accurate on-site assessment, as well as expertise in the immediate response components (triage, evacuation, etc) is critical.

The first step to achieving a disaster response capability is the engagement of Governments in the institution of appropriate EMS Systems that will have not only the capability but also the responsibility for local/regional medical participation into the overall management of a disaster. This means that each system and each hospital should develop their own planning and also gain necessary skills. At the same time, they should establish appropriate coordination with the other agencies involved in the response.

Although improvisation may always have a role at the scene, each agency should imagine disaster situations and pre-plan the appropriate response. Such response, however, should be based upon routine operations, since it is known that distress situations lead the personnel to act automatically. Plans should be simple and flexible in order to allow a phased response according to the type and the extent of the disaster.

However, experience has shown that a perfect linkage among the agencies responsible for the above-mentioned activities is found to be almost impossible. It is our belief that only accurate studies and discussions among the involved agencies (police, fire departments, mass media, regional authority) may lead to adequate pre-planning with a view to the overall integration of emergency medical services into the global disaster response.

Civil military medical cooperation should also be considered in planning response, mainly on a regional/national level.

The Civil Defense Agency will be the most high level appropriate authority in the overall response of the community to a disaster.

2. SPECIFIC ISSUES

Disaster planning must be considered in regional/national and in prehospital/in-hospital levels.

(a) Pre-hospital/In-hospital Planning

For approaching this issue, it seems wise to start with in-hospital plans. As mentioned before, the first step should be to determine the disruption ratio, or in other words, how a hospital should deal with overload. This can then be tied into plans for the mobilization of the prehospital EMS System.

Possible disruption of communications, transportation and personnel availability should also be considered. Special attention should be given to stock supplies, equipment and facilities. This means that planning needs to be conditioned on the vulnerability of the system. In-hospital disaster planning is time-consuming and unpopular. On the other hand, personnel under stress situations have a general tendency to work according to the routine procedures. This justifies to have simple and flexible emergency therapeutic protocols, the implementation of which will be the basis for planning.

Within hospitals there should exist an established administrative pattern, including the definition of who has the authority to declare a state of disaster and of a clear hierarchy chain. The duties of the administrator or chief of staff as well as those of the hospital staff (physicians, nurses, paramedics) should be clearly defined.

The hospital disaster plan should incorporate three main components:

(i) medical management of casualties;
(ii) staff alert, recall and deployment
(iii) information, control and communications

The essential characteristic of hospital response planning is, therefore, its capability of providing a sudden increase in emergency services. The plan for small catastrophes is expanded in major disasters, through a phased mobilization of more personnel and equipment, rather than through other, more specific alterations.

For this purpose each hospital should have an appropriate Disaster Manual, easily identifiable, and containing brief summary of policies and procedures, followed by detailed annexes.

In the community, several agencies should be involved in local disaster planning, such as the police, fire departments, EMS System, transport authority, communications. Public information media have a very relevant role, disseminating adequate information in order to avoid panic and help the population, spreading messages from health authorities, etc. Each agency should have responsibility and authority assigned by region and by function.

(b) Regional/National Planning

From the local plans can evolve regional and national plans, with arrangements for mutual aid, including resources from outside the disaster area.

In these cases, attention should be first given to the special characteristics of the area under consideration. It is necessary to collect the best available geographic and demographic data and then estimate the probability of specific disaster situations that the history of the region may identify as potential hazards, not only natural disasters but also the consequences of industrial and technological accidents or civil unrest.

Specific attention should be given to:

(i) Characteristics of each type of potential disaster;
(ii) Estimate of the number and severity of expected casualties;
(iii) Available warning systems;
(iv) Expected time lag of information transmission;
(v) Location and potential mobility of available resources.

The plans should be developed with the basis on such forecasting and should require pre-testing through rehearsals and drills. Periodic appraisals of available resources and needs, for augmentation, relocation, and modernization are required.

At regional/national planning, and even at an international level of mutual aid agreements, it has been recognized that only a wellidentified, authoritative coordinating body involving all agencies will be the solution for the majority of the problems concerning the limitation of efficiency and effectiveness of the community counteraction to disaster.

Within the general medical response planning, some specific points and strategic aspects also should be considered:

(i) The need for a basic organization that should be the most effective way of facing a disaster. Such objective will be accomplished through the implementation of EMS Systems;

(ii) Identification and coordination of all possible resources is imperative for disaster planning;

(iii) The exchange of information on past disaster experiences should be increased. Data banks are needed;

(iv) One of the rolls of Preventive Medicine should be the institution of conditions for surveillance of diseases that are endemic in a given area, but may increase in incidence following a disaster situation;

(v) Effort for correct on-site assessment should be attempted as first priority in the field;

(vi) Continued study and research on the impact of several types of disasters upon the body and the mind should be implemented;

(vii) Medico-legal aspects, concerning not only the problem of the identification of the victim, but also some legal aspects of emergency care as well as the forensic research of the pathologist, should be considered;

(viii) Psychological and Social Welfare problems, namely involving attempts at adaptation, defense mechanisms and new emotional situations should be faced;

(ix) Military command "know-how" through close medical cooperation is relevant on effectiveness of civil command chain;

(x) Education and training in the new dimension of Disaster Medicine need to be taken into account.

EDUCATION AND TRAINING

In this field, three major issues should be approached: team-work, the management of change, the technological advance and the environment.

Preparedness to face these aspects of disaster response should begin at a school level, mainly in health schools, according to the different degrees of education.

Public information on first aid and safety rules are first steps towards self-help in the community. The voluntary aid organizations have here a relevant role. On the other hand, campaigns on the mass media are valuable to increase awareness and understanding.

Some technical schools and activities, such as factories of chemicals and weapons, as well as those people involved in the transportation of hazardous materials, should be concerned with education and training adequate to risk of disaster.

Health schools, mainly Medical College, and also Nursing and Paramedic schools, should be the core of commitment in Disaster Medicine education, both in the technical and social fields. However, this doesn't mean specialization, but discussion and information on well defined notions, including basic aspects of accidents and trauma, medical emergencies, toxicologic and psychiatric emergencies under a disaster point of view. Family doctors living at the disaster area, if trained in basic life support and triage skills, and with knowledge of the correct methodology of disaster notification, no doubt have a very important role before the arrival of the specialized rescue teams at the scene.

Training of the response system to disaster is really the main issue.

As mentioned before, the best preparedness at the level of health structures is based upon the implementation of the routine emergency operations of a well established Emergency Medical Services System, according to simple and flexible plans. Each hospital, each system should develop appropriate training programs, based upon on their own disaster plans.

On the other hand, similar programs should be carried out in cooperation with all agencies involved, following an overall realistic plan. These drills should essentially take into account the risks of natural disasters (earthquakes, floods, tidal waves, volcanic eruptions) and risks of technological accidents (chemical intoxications, industrial explosions, large fires, radioactive contaminations, air, road and major water incidents).

Special attention should be given to the critical aspects of joint exercises, as far as command, control and coordination are concerned. Civil-Military cooperation certainly has an important role in this field.

TEACHING AND TRAINING IN EMERGENCY AND DISASTER MEDICINE

Corrado Manni, M.D., Professor
Director, Institute of Anaesthesiology and
Intensive Care Medicine
Catholic University of Sacred Heart - Rome - Italy

The establishment of different programs aimed at teaching Emergency and Disaster Medicine must be based on the observation that these disciplines present, apart from their common features, many differences, especially in terms of strategies, tactics, techniques and ethical aspects of first aid.

The strategies, in fact, are very dissimilar: Emergency Medicine is practiced every day in the context of well-defined, proven structures; Disaster Medicine, on the other hand, takes place in much more complex and, almost always, unforeseen conditions, using improvised support structures, or at least structures that have been hastily put together.

As far as tactics go, there certainly exists some common ground between the two disciplines. For example: the necessity of rapid intervention; the correct use of telecommunications; triage; finding out which medical centers have the best facilities for dealing with that type of pathology. At the same time, Emergency Medicine does not include, for example, the implementation of plans for evacuation or triage on a large scale.

Moreover, the specialist in Emergency Medicine is usually called on to assist in cases within the hospital, while in Disaster Medicine many of the operations take place on the spot with whatever means are available.

The first aid techniques are similar, but are put into practice in a more simplified, standardized way when faced with a calamity of one kind or another.

Notable differences also arise concerning the deontological and ethical norms of medical assistance: Emergency Medicine is, in fact, aimed at the individual, while Disaster Medicine is aimed at providing assistance to entire populations. The latter presupposes therefore the interest of the whole over that of the individual.

Thus, whenever setting up programs for the training and teaching of "Emergency and Disaster Medicine," it is necessary to answer two fundamental questions:

- Whom to teach;
- What to teach.

Health and Medical Aspects of Disaster Preparedness
Edited by J.C. Duffy
Plenum Press, New York, 1990

WHOM TO TEACH

Training and refresher courses in Emergency and Disaster Medicine are not only for doctors and medical personnel, but also for other professionals and the average citizen; anyone, in fact, can find themselves involved in a health emergency and called on to provide the first decisive assistance or to collaborate later on with medical experts.

Naturally, such courses will vary in content depending on the audience they are designed for.

Educating the Entire Population

The training of large segments of the population should have as its primary goal the teaching of the most basic first aid measures aimed at reviving and/or maintaining vital functions.

The experience of Intensive Care Units in the past few years shows that the prognosis for patients who suffer a sudden loss of conscience or cardio-respiratory arrest is in direct relation to the immediate implementation of simple therapeutic actions, such as keeping air passages open, using External Cardiac Massage, or employing mouth-to-mouth resuscitation.

It is the right and duty of everyone to know these therapeutic procedures; any delay in using them, even for just 2-3 minutes, means a complete change in the outcome of the pathology and renders useless future, usually futile, assistance.

The present situation is that, faced with an emergency situation of this kind, the average person, not knowing what to do, refrains from providing any kind of aid. Worse still, attempts of some form of assistance which not only might <u>not</u> benefit the patient, but can, in some cases, actually cause serious and irreversible damage; for example, placing the patient in a sitting position or trying to administer liquids by mouth.

Anyone who has seen a traffic accident will have been aware that the inherent dramatic force of the incident is increased enormously by the impossibility of providing immediate, adequate aid.

In most cases, spectators who have happened on to the scene do not know what to do and wait helplessly for the arrival of medical professionals. Unfortunately, the prognosis of an acute pathology is directly related to the time before assistance is administered and not just to the quality of the assistance. If those passers-by knew a few simple operational procedures they would be able to recognize and stop an external hemorrhage, place the injured person in the correct position so as to prevent the onset of shock, or remove any obstructions from the upper respiratory passages of an unconscious victim.

If known, these procedures can be carried out by anyone; their immediate implementation allows the victim to rapidly overcome any critical situation. It would be opportune therefore to put into place large scale programs for teaching first aid.

Training programs are costly in terms of personnel, time and money, but epidemiological data justify their implementation; in fact, the number of accidental, unforeseen deaths (by trauma, poisoning, etc.) is so disproportionately high that a basic knowledge of the first steps to take in aiding a victim can dramatically increase the rate of survival.

The objectives of a beginner's course in cardiorespiratory care can be summed up in the following points: a) to recognize the need for resuscitation, b) to recognize the need for urgent action c) to begin a correct series of actions and d) to acquire a permanent "hands on" knowledge through the use of various didactic materials such as manuals, audiovisual aids, mannequins and computerized simulators that permit a valuable interaction with the subject.

Educating Volunteers

Constituting a spontaneous form of public mobilization which thus expresses their solidarity with victims in the disaster area, volunteers can play a decisive role in emergency situations and, above all, during serious calamities. This holds true, however, only if good will and enthusiasm can be combined with preparation, professionalism and discipline. Anything less than this and the work of volunteers can be more damaging and dangerous than useful, as experience has shown during several recent natural disasters. On the other hand, if well-prepared, volunteers could carry out a number of different tasks, such as:

1) Collaborating in a program of health education for the general population or in special cases, with the goal of preventing or mitigating the effects of catastrophic events.

2) Participating in the realization of specific programs of intervention in collaboration with officially licensed first aid centers.

3) Coordinating the immediate mobilization and intervention of other citizens during the initial phases of a disaster.

4) Providing first aid to victims while waiting for professional help to arrive.

Educating Personnel from Other Services

All members of the police force, firefighters, crews on boats and planes, airport employees, factory and hotel workers should receive training in basic first aid and in particular in cardiocirculatory resuscitation. Moreover, they should be aware of all emergency plans which refer to the places where they work and they should be able to compile a report on a disaster which contains fundamental information on the number of wounded, the types of injuries and any other information helpful in providing ideal assistance proportionate to the true needs of the situation.

Educating Nursing Personnel

Every emergency plan provides for the use of nursing personnel in providing health assistance and their utility is beyond question. Apart from their invaluable role in giving medical assistance, they are also able to lend important moral support to victims of a disaster as well as their family and friends. Nursing staff thus needs special training with particular emphasis on the ability to lead and on the difficulties they can face in carrying out their professional activity "on the spot" and in difficult conditions.

Educating Personnel from Mobile and Units

These are the people who usually find themselves involved in emergency situations and who should already possess sufficient knowledge for dealing with critical pathologies.

Ambulance teams, mobile intensive care units and helicopter ambulance squads should take courses emphasizing triage, the risks connected with subjective emotional factors, the danger of fatigue and the variety of possible environmental conditions they may encounter at the site of a disaster.

Very often, in fact, health care personnel possess the knowledge and experience necessary to face a "mini-emergency", but are unprepared to face a large scale disaster.

Educating specialists in Emergency and Disaster Medicine

Emergency Health Services should make sure of specialists specifically prepared for and able to intervene in each phase of a rescue operation.

The first phase includes recognizing and delineating the devastated area. The medical specialist then cooperates with rescue teams already on the spot in counting the victims and determining the predominant health needs so as to aid in a qualitative way later assistance. During the evacuation of the wounded it is up to the specialist to choose the most ideal means of transport according to the victims' condition. The specialist must also establish the priority in the evacuation.

The second phase includes triage and the organization of a first aid center; the role of the doctor in this case is essential but also very difficult. He must take an active part in the initial treatment of the victims (infusions, artificial respiration, sedation, other specific treatments).

During the third phase, the large scale evacuation of the victims to hospital, the medical specialist must continue to oversee operations and provide medical assistance.

The skills necessary for training a capable expert in Emergency and Disaster Medicine are many.

In particular: the expert must be ready to make a snap decision on unusual or very rare pathologies: radiation sickness, chemical burns, mass poisonings, panic.

As far as techniques go, the expert must know simplified and standardized methods relative to the administration of medicines, to respiratory assistance and to sedation.

Other techniques too, such as the extrication of victims and the transmission of information by radio, must also be perfectly understood.

Unfortunately, many universities still do not have specific courses in Emergency and Disaster Medicine. The training of medical personnel occurs almost exclusively through post-university training and refresher courses.

WHAT TO TEACH

It is possible to put forth a broad outline of both the programs to teach and the means with which to teach them.

The subjects of these programs can be divided into several basic groups:

1) Cardiorespiratory Resuscitation (CPR)

Everyone should be able to diagnose a cardiorespiratory arrest and execute three basic maneuvers aimed at sustaining vital functions: keeping the air passages open; mouth-to-mouth resuscitation; external heart massage.

Quickly carrying out these relatively simple maneuvers protects the integrity of the central nervous system even for long periods until the arrival of medical professionals who will then look after the victim.

2) The first steps for aiding the Traumatized Patient

The continual rise in the number of traffic accidents places before us each day the problem of dealing with a patient suffering from multiple injuries. Anyone should be able to place the subject in the correct position, staunch any external hemorrhage without causing further injuries (ischemia, anoxia), and move the patient from the site of the incident to a means of transport.

3) Aiding an Unconscious Patient

It is absurd that a simple "phlebotomy" could result in death. Unfortunately it happens more often than one would think, as well both due to a lack of assistance and to assistance improperly administered by inexperienced rescuers.

Trying to place an unconscious person into a sitting position or just to try and raise the person's head could cause the flow of blood to the brain to be reduced so much that it causes death; even more foolhardy are the attempts frequently observed, to make the unconscious patient drink liquids; the result is inhalation and the upper obstruction of the respiratory tracts.

Even if carried out through different programs, the general populace must be taught the aforementioned diagnostic-therapeutic techniques.

The basic ideas can be put across through the press and the usual audio-visual means (television, radio, cinema, theater). It should be simple information, immediate, repeated periodically, so that it clearly indicates what must be done and, above all, what must not be done.

A more complete and possibly theoretic-practical example can be made regarding the schools. Direct teaching presents unarguable advantages and only through the teacher-student exchange can doubts be resolved and the subject thoroughly covered.

Finally, for those groups of people who are frequently involved in rescue operations (police, firefighters, etc.) it is necessary to increase the number of advanced courses with relative examinations and periodic refresher seminars.

The medical emergency, as experience in many different nations has shown, would undoubtedly benefit from these suggestions both in "mini-emergencies" as well as in "maxi-emergencies."

It is above all in the latter case, when the victim-rescuer proportion is so high as to frustrate any operation, that the ability to receive useful assistance from the general public becomes the only way to reduce to minimum the number of injuries.

4) Triage

Knowledge of triage techniques is generally not needed in operations that take place on a day-to-day basis because those "mini-emergencies" usually involve a limited number of victims.

On the other hand, when faced with a large scale disaster the rescuers' first task is to identify the victims with life-threatening wounds who need immediate treatment and evacuation. Even well-trained nursing personnel are able to perform these operations while awaiting the arrival of the doctor.

The victims must be rapidly classified into four categories:

EE (Extreme emergency) = evacuation impossible, needs immediate treatment.
E1 (serious) = immediate evacuation after vital functions stabilized.
E2 (less serious) = delayed evacuation
E3 (light wounds) = no urgent treatment needed.

Training in triage techniques can be carried out through the use of practice exercises. The instructors should simulate the wounds which occur in disasters the class is being taught about (for example: an airplane crash or terrorist attack).

Triage training can also be done by using specific exercises: after having given the students a list of wounds relative to a certain number of wounded, and after having supplied them with detailed information on the available personnel and equipment, the students must classify the victims according to priority, giving reasons for their choices.

5) Techniques relative to rescue work outside the hospital

The objective of this training must be to give rescue workers practice in working outside the hospital's walls. Very often in fact, health workers have very little experience working outside the typical, well-equipped hospital, with its carefully ordered atmosphere and with all the necessary means at one's fingertips; yet

in the typical disaster situation one must work at the scene of the incident.

Equipment is therefore limited to the minimum that can be transported; ideal working conditions do not exist and the people available to assist may be neither willing nor able to work in such conditions.

Training in using a reduced amount of equipment can be acquired by working with rescue teams in ambulances, at dangerous sporting events (car races, rallies, marathons), and in situations where large numbers of people are gathered.

Beyond this, many disasters come about due to environmental pollution. Rescue workers can therefore be asked to work in dangerous conditions. In such situations it is necessary to wear special protective clothing. Thus, there should be training as to their use especially for facing situations in which one is exposed to toxic chemical substances or to nuclear radiation.

Finally, rescue workers should be familiar with decontamination procedures. Everyone should be aware of the symptoms of overexposure, which could also strike rescuers.

6) Running Rescue Operations

Managing rescue operations at a disaster requires an efficient system of administration. Health workers, maintaining their autonomy as far as the medical aspects of the victims' treatment go, must be prepared to follow the orders given by personnel from other services such as: firefighters, demolition experts, police and military authorities.

7) Ethical and Deontological Problems

During a disaster, rescue workers--and in particular doctors--must be able to deal with complex ethical and deontological problems.

During everyday emergencies they are used to being called on to attempt to save the life of a single patient even in desperate conditions; on the other hand during a disaster, they could find themselves in a situation in which this type of victim must be passed over in order to dedicate more time to a patient with better chances for survival.

8) Rescue Techniques

During rescue operations, medical personnel must be prepared to be flexible with regard to their own fields of specialization. That means that every doctor should be trained in basic resuscitation procedures and in controlling hemorrhages; the doctor should be able to prepare a main blood passageway to carry out a rapid transfusion, to insert a thoracic drain, to immobilize a fracture of the spinal column, and to know how to treat serious burns.

It is essential, therefore, that doctors be able to work outside the boundaries of their own particular field.

Intensive therapy wards and Intensive Care Units, operating halls and emergency rooms are the ideal places for gaining this kind of experience.

9) Communications

In many disaster situations the problem of difficult communications arises: communications among rescue workers, communications between the hospital and the disaster site, and, at times, even communications with the hospital itself.

Doctors and medical personnel therefore need to have basic training in the use of radio equipment and other means of communication.

Such training can be found at ambulance centers, with the coast guard or in flight schools.

10) Mass Media

Means of communicating with the mass media are essential in managing rescue operations during a catastrophe. News bulletins to the press should be given out only by one authorized source who is trained in media relations. Such a source should be represented by doctors specialized in Emergency and Disaster Medicine.

It is imperative that no one at the scene of the incident gives interviews or expounds his or her own personal view of the situation. That usually causes useless and even dangerous alarm.

It is essential as well to critically examine and, if necessary rectify, the reports and information which the media gives on the incident. Indeed, the principal objective of the press is to make news and thus situations are presented which often do not correspond to reality.

PSYCHOLOGICAL ASPECTS

Rescue workers must be aware that in facing a disastrous event, they can become involved psychically, and that can have negative consequences on their behavior and on their efficiency.

Also, a slow response in the face of such a catastrophe can be due in part to the effect of surprise when suddenly confronted with an unexpected event. From this point of view it is rather difficult to advise training since few of us know beforehand our own particular type of reaction when faced with a real life situation.

But this specific area, simulations of a disaster scenario can be very useful. In fact, what prevails in a disaster situation is panic, fear, the uncertainty over what the best action is; in many disasters, panic can cause more damage than the incident itself.

The description of disaster scenarios can thus help participants in training courses to become used to conditions which can occur during a catastrophe. This can contribute to reducing the effect of surprise, panic, and the sense of helplessness which so often take over in these situations. Films, documentaries and photographs can be very useful in describing disaster scenarios and giving to participants in a course an overall picture of the effects a disaster can cause.

From the didactic point of view, descriptions of previous natural disasters and the way in which citizens and rescue organizations reacted can also be very useful.

During training it is also important to remember that no one is indispensable and that fatigue hits everyone, so no one in a disaster operation should try to stay on the job beyond his or her own limits. There is no place for pride in these situations and everyone must be ready to give up his or her place to a colleague at the opportune moment.

TYPES OF DISASTERS AND SPECIFIC TRAINING PROBLEMS

To carry out an adequate training program it is best to classify disasters in two main categories: for each type, a specific preparation is necessary.

The first type is the disaster which takes place in an industrialized country where there already exist sufficient means and qualified personnel for undertaking rescue operations. The other type is the disaster which takes place in a developing country where, due to the scarcity of resources, infrastructures and other means, the death and injury rate can be disproportionately high. In this case any small difficulty could be enough to provoke disastrous results if there already exists a chronic health care situation.

A) MANAGING DISASTERS IN INDUSTRIALIZED COUNTRIES

Many countries are currently equipped with efficient Emergency Health Services which are able to meet daily calamities as well as large scale disasters. These nations possess the ideal means of mobile rescue and a network of hospitals able to offer a wide range of specialized medical treatment. With these means it is possible to handle without great difficulty the majority of small scale disasters, both natural as well as man-made. Still, it is necessary to supply specific training aimed at perfecting the care and treatment of a large number of patients. Such training would take place however, without neglecting the daily requests for assistance.

It is opportune to recall that a disaster can also involve the structures of the hospital itself, as in the case of the earthquakes.

In such circumstances, cool heads and professionalism must prevail while awaiting the rapid evacuation of the hospital.

The medical treatments which must be carried out on a large number of patients really do not differ much from those which are performed on a daily basis. There are, however, certain supplementary actions which can be performed and several modifications of the standard therapeutic protocol which can help to provide better care for a large number of victims.

The entire personnel of the hospital should be aware of emergency plans and there should be periodic practice simulations organized to familiarize the personnel with the various situations which could occur in a hospital.

Administrative personnel should be trained in dealing with the media, with the police, and should be taught how to interpret medical bulletins.

B) MANAGING DISASTERS IN DEVELOPING COUNTRIES

In developing countries, the loss of human life is often all out of proportion with respect to the disaster; and long-term, international assistance is frequently necessary after a catastrophe.

Procedures regarding international cooperation should therefore be well-known to experts in Emergency and Disaster Medicine.

The essential requirements for undertaking an effective rescue operation in a developing country are diplomacy and tolerance combined with quality administrative management, with a didactic capacity and a knowledge of the structures available on the site. Knowledge of the language is another important requirement which can be overcome with the help of interpreters.

Volunteers must be certain to be in good health and prepared to live in primitive conditions. They will have to make sure they are protected against whatever infectious diseases may be prevalent in the area and should carry with them their own personal supply of medicines. A sick rescue worker would only be a further obstacle to the other workers. Everyone who volunteers to work in a developing country in a disaster situation should know mass vaccination procedures.

Since chronic malnutrition is frequently present in these countries and is in fact one of the greatest problems, all volunteers should be able to treat this particular pathological state. Rehydration and xxrenteral feeding could be necessary in the worst cases but this procedure should be employed only if it is possible to use a vein without risking infection.

Rescue workers should also leave a disaster zone only after having passed on at least part of their experience to the local residents. Training and educating the resident population is even more valuable than individual clinical care, provided the two aspects are closely correlated.

Upon returning from an operation, the doctor, nurse or technician will have an enhanced knowledge and experience that should be passed on to others through published articles and conferences. They will be the ones who know best the problems and needs of an affected zone and will therefore be best able to indicate the most useful means that should be sent.

TRAINING AND REFRESHER COURSES

To train qualified specialists in disaster medicine it is necessary to set up education and training courses which, as has already been noted, are very often not included in average medical curriculums. The training should be of a theoretical-practical nature, and should be given by people with personal experience in managing disasters.

Above all, the courses should deal with those aspects which differentiate Disaster Medicine from other branches of medicine. Also, if the practical exercises are to be effective, they must be carried out using realistic simulations and scenarios, and using numerous victims represented by mannequins or, better yet, other volunteers.

An example of a course in Disaster Medicine is the one organized by SAMU 94 of Paris, which has been held twice a year since 1981. In each session 40 students are accepted from all over France as well as from abroad. The students are civilians, general practitioners, or specialists (mainly in Anaesthesiology and Intensive Care). In some cases they are military doctors or personnel attached to fire departments.

The theoretical program covers 80 hours which are subdivided as follows:

- 2 hours introduction on the history of disasters and the different types of disasters.

- 13 hours dedicated to strategy and in particular to evaluating national and international emergency plans.

- 23 hours given over to the tactics and logistics of triage, means of telecommunications, evacuation procedures, field hospital, hygiene, resupplying foodstuffs and legal questions.

- 10 hours to removing and extricating victims and providing for their initial treatment.

- 28 hours dealing with the different types of pathologies one can come across in a disaster situation: wounds resulting from a crushing blow, exposure to gas or cold, burns, drownings, explosions or wounds caused by firearms, radioactive contamination, panic, as well as craniofacial, thoracic, abdominal and vascular injuries.

The practical training takes place at the end of each course through the collaboration of the army's health corps.

The principle aim of this course is to train doctors so that they might know better how to act in an emergency situation and might be better able to take part, with discipline and efficiency, in the various phases of a rescue operation. The diploma in Disaster Medicine is granted only to those who have shown a solid theoretical knowledge and have passed certain tests given during the practical exercises.

Another organization which deals specifically with preparation and training in Catastrophe Medicine is the European Center for Catastrophe Medicine (CEMEC: Centro Europeo per la Medicine delle Catastrofi), which was founded in San Marino in 1986 under the auspices of the Council of Europe. The goal of CEMEC is to reduce the effects of both technological and natural catastrophes through research, studies, training courses and international and interregional exchanges, especially among the various European countries.

CEMEC works in close collaboration with the Council of Europe, the World Health Organization (WHO) and the Office of the United Nations Disaster Relief Coordinator (UNDRO), bringing its own scientific and educational contribution to the fight against the suffering and devastation caused by catastrophes.

Each year it organizes training courses in Catastrophe Medicine. These courses are open to medical personnel, nurses, volunteer rescue workers, and Civil Defense terms.

Courses organized for three weeks of training deal with the following themes: "Early health assistance measures in large-scale emergencies: at the site and during transport"; "Burns over a large area, organization of aid"; "Managing the crisis: information and communications: the role of the mass media."

The subjects which will be dealt with during the first course are the following:

1) Cerebral and cardio-respiratory resuscitation: first and second phase
2) Specific first aid operations
3) Pain therapy
4) Shock
5) Respiratory distress syndrome(ARDS).
6) Crush syndrome
7) Acute renal insufficiency
8) Diagnosis and therapy for arrhythmia
9) Emergency toxicology
10) Radiation catastrophes
11) Feeding in catastrophes
12) Exercises: techniques of cardio-respiratory resuscitation, means of first aid
13) Audio-visual documentation

The subjects of the second course will be the following:

1) Catastrophes caused by fire
2) Medico-surgical therapy and organization for burns
3) Psychological effects of burns over a large area
4) Burns caused by toxic substances
5) Nuclear disasters
6) International aid to affected areas
7) The United Nations regional coordinating office
8) The Red Cross and Non-Governmental Organizations in disasters
9) International transportation of the wounded
10) Provisions and logistics
11) International problems

And finally, the subjects which will be dealt with in the third week:

1) The role of the mass media in catastrophes
2) At whom it is aimed
3) The Protagonists
4) Means of spreading information
5) Education
6) Training the public
7) General principles in preparing for and intervening in catastrophes
8) Psychological aspects
9) Epidemiology
10) Specific psycho-social actions for the victims and for rescue workers
11) Evaluating needs in relation to the affected community
12) Planning intervention

If we have set down in detail the program of these courses it is because in this way we can best answer the question "what to teach" within the limits of a discipline, "Disaster Medicine," which is still evolving and searching for a specific identity.

A PLANNING MODEL FOR DISASTER RESPONSE

Howard R. Champion, M.D., Chief, Trauma Service

Director, Surgical and Critical Care Service
The Washington Hospital Center
Washington, D.C.

INTRODUCTION

Two major characteristics of disaster complicate man's ability to respond to them effectively. First, they happen with little or no warning, and second, disasters are unique in time and place. Therefore, to best address a planning model that provides a timely and efficient approach to response, it is necessary to review the experiences of previous actual incidences, extract the common elements, and evaluate the response performance. Using this process, the following model was developed.

The first step in disaster planning involves a clear understanding of the nature and characteristics of disasters. A definition and classification of disasters is presented in Exhibit 1.

TYPE OF RESPONSE

The area encompassed by the disaster, indicates which of several types of response classifications is appropriate. There are multiple layers of responses to disasters which can be classified by the area encompassed by the disaster. These response types are:

Institutional
Local
Subregional
Regional
State or National

DEFINITION AND CLASSIFICATION OF DISASTERS

Definitio: A disaster is a serious disruption to life, public, order, security or safety that arises with little or no warning. It threatens or causes death or injury to a number of public services operating under normal conditions, and thus requires special mobilization of those services.

Classification: A disaster should be classified in a manner which will enable the incident commander to request specific types and levels of response. Classification must describe the nature and extent of the problem.

Health and Medical Aspects of Disaster Preparedness
Edited by J.C. Duffy
Plenum Press, New York, 1990

Nature: Disasters can be simple (a railway accident) or compound (an earthquake). Confrontation disasters are those that are associated with war or terrorist activities. Natural disasters include floods, earthquakes, epidemics and famine. Technological disasters result from the failure of increasingly complex systems used to support society or personnel who operate them. Technological disasters may include peace time chemical or radiation exposure, building, or bridge or other structural collapse, fire, and transport system accidents involving aircraft, ships, trains or motor vehicles.

Extent: The extent estimate of the number of victims killed or injured, or at risk of death or injury, thus identifying in general the level of regional response (See Exhibit 1).

Not all disasters involve a threat to or loss of life and consequently must be described in terms other than those given here, e.g., acreage involved in fire, potential threat to life, radiation exposure.

Exhibit 1

Level	Killed/Injured		Requiring Hospitalization	RESPONSE
Minor	Up to 25	and /or	Up to 10	Local jurisdiction only, with sub-regional notification
Moderate	Over 25 Up to 100	and /or	Over 10 Up to 50	Subregional plus regional alert, including regional Trauma Centers
Major	Over 00- Up to 1,000	and /or	Over 50 Up to 250	Regional response with extra-regional states and military alerted

CLEARLY IT IS THE RESPONSIBILITY OF THE MOST SENIOR LOCAL AUTHORITY AT THE SITE OF A DISASTER TO DETERMINE INITIALLY THE NATURE AND EXTENT OF THE DISASTER, SO THAT AN APPROPRIATE DISASTER RESPONSE CAN BE INITIATED.

As Exhibit 1 indicates, the number and condition of disaster victims are the major determinants for selecting the type of response needed to handle the disaster. A more complex disaster requires a larger number and variation of response resources.

Most minor disasters easily can be handled without extending the emergency response beyond a single local jurisdiction. A moderate disaster often requires selective augmentation of local capabilities with additional vehicles and facilities. The level of the problem should dictate the level of the response. Between a minor and a moderate disaster a sensible response is to provide triage treatment teams from regional hospitals with trauma centers and to send patients both to these institutions and to the local hospitals close to the disaster. Clearly, when a major disaster occurs, every hospital and facility within a region will be incorporated into the disaster. Coordinating the components of a regional disaster response to a moderate level disaster requires specific planning and testing above and beyond that for a local disaster response.

COMPONENTS OF A PLANNING MODEL

The components of a planning model include but are not limited to: a plan, jurisdictional and respondent Mutual Aid Agreements, training and human resource development, resource identification, response process, geographic and cultural address, and post disaster evaluation.

THE PLAN

There are three major levels of disaster response: (1) the internal hospital (institutional) level; (2) the local level involving fire, police, and rescue operations, and resource associate hospitals; and (3) the regional level, requiring multijurisdictional cooperation and coordination. Disaster plans must be generated from all levels, and coordination of intent and activity must be ensured. All disaster plans and response must have the following general characteristics.

1. The plan must be simple and must function as a natural outgrowth to daily operational systems. When responding to the crisis situation, individuals perform best at those tasks which they are capable of doing and react in a manner that is most suited to their training and background.

2. The response must integrate all aspects of existing emergency medical services (EMS). Given that the disaster response is based on day-to-day operations and incorporates all ongoing operations in manner reflecting their normal relationships, the scope of the disaster response can be flexible and open-ended.

3. The disaster response must be managed by intelligent, well trained individuals who can adapt the response to the various circumstances that may be encountered. Flexibility is essential, since no two disasters are exactly alike.

4. The planned disaster response must be written concisely and simply and posted in easily available areas. An internal hospital telephone directory containing a one-page streamlined summary of a disaster response, and a "chest sheet" on the wall of the regional dispatch center the response to be initiated while a manual provides the details.

5. The disaster response must be rehearsed in its entirety around specific scenarios.

MUTUAL AID AGREEMENTS

Mutual Aid Agreements serve to facilitate the response, particularly in regional disasters, when multiple agencies, and respondents, etc., must be mobilized. Through these agreements and their subsequent coordination of activities, duplication or neglect of response procedures is avoided. Cooperation of the multi-disciplines hopefully expedites response procedures and avoids unnecessary bureaucratic delays.

The agreements should contain procedural as well as operational aspects of response, specifically:

- delineation of the authority of participating bodies in the event of an emergency

- provision for the delegation of responsibility under Mutual Aid; and

- definition of the authority of either the police chief or fire chief of the requesting jurisdiction when requesting aid under the terms of either the Policy or Fire/Rescue Mutual Aid Agreements.

TRAINING AND HUMAN RESOURCE MANPOWER DEVELOPMENT

The objective of Training and Human Resource development is to provide public safety personnel with the skill, knowledge, and expertise to respond rapidly, effectively and appropriately to disasters in the area. Training and familiarization programs are essential to improving disaster response. Public safety agencies can strengthen the ability to respond to disasters by instituting multi-disciplinary training efforts. Often, utilizing the wealth of resources in the region-experienced personnel and facilities may assist in multidisciplinary training.

It is recommended that any disaster response planning model contains a training and human resource development component which would:

- Conduct periodic and regular regionwide disaster drills around specific scenarios.

- Provide debriefings and evaluations for disaster response personnel after a disaster drill or actual response.

- Institute a familiarization program for Command Physicians and for physicians forming Physicians Response Teams from the designated regional Trauma Centers.

RESPONSE IDENTIFICATION

A planning model must identify and list specialized pre-hospital resources which include vehicles and extracting equipment, personnel, and specialized communication capability. (See Exhibits 2, 3, 4).

The purpose of cataloging these resources and itemizing their respective capabilities is two-fold. First, it provides a quick reference to the distribution and location of resources. Secondly, it allows for easy assessment of gaps in resource capability. A similar matrix may be developed for designated trauma centers and hospitals in the region.

RESPONSE PROCESS

INITIAL DISASTER RESPONSE AT THE SCENE

Word of a disaster reaches the appropriate resources in many ways. Misrepresentations may be expressed in communications by shocked citizens who cannot believe that they are part of the scene unfolding before them. It is likely that a 10 to 15 minute delay may exist when relaying timely, accurate information. In fact, in natural disasters, communications may be totally obliterated, as was the experience in the Japanese earthquakes of the 1970s. As a result, their response relied on local activities without the benefit of regional coordination.

The first public service responder at the scene should assess the extent and nature of the disaster and promptly report the following to the Communications and Dispatch Center so that resources can be mobilized: (1) the nature of the disaster; (2) an estimate of the number of casualties and their severity; and (3) the accessibility of the scene.

After advising the Dispatch Center of these findings, the senior medically trained individual, usually an emergency medical technician (EMT), assumes command at the scene until fire and rescue personnel arrive. During this interval, the EMT explores the disaster area, identifying the pockets of casualties and estimating the number of rescue-triage teams that will be required.

The fire department, the police, and ambulance personnel should be dispatched to the scene. In addition to extinguishing and preventing fires, the fire department is responsible for securing and maintaining safety at the disaster scene and assessing the risks involved in the disaster response. Also, the fire department is involved in the rescue operation and is responsible for the mobilization of auxiliary resources.

The police are responsible for maintaining the perimeter and integrity of the disaster site and for ensuring unencumbered access and egress for EMS personnel when the area surrounding the disaster become crowded. Ambulance personnel perform primary and secondary triage and treatment and transport victims to designated hospitals.

Authority relationships at the disaster site are essential to effective management. Usually, the senior fire department official takes charge. Recognition of the fire department, police, and EMS personnel is essential. The outer layer of protective clothing should be color-coded for identification, e.g., red for fire and blue for EMS, since arm bands are not adequate.

COMMAND AND COMMUNICATION

Once a disaster has been identified, a command and communication post should be established at the scene as rapidly as possible. This command post should be close to the disaster to receive stretcher-carried victims, yet remote enough to safely control major routes of access and egress. Also, this command post can serve as a secondary triage and evacuation area. The functions of the command center are as follows:

COMMAND. Successful response to a disaster depends heavily on human response to an authority figure. The post must be established with this awareness and with a clear view to exercise command and to be seen as exercising command. To this end, command should be highly visible so that personnel responding to the disaster can identify the command, and then promptly report and receive instruction.

COMMUNICATION. Information communicated to the Dispatch Center identifies the scope and nature of the disaster and the needed level of response. Corresponding regional mobilization from the Dispatch Center confirms the command structure and its location at the disaster site (Figure 1). In major disasters, hospital-to-ambulance medical communications usually should be curtailed, and paramedics and other physician extenders should function under disaster protocol or the direct orders of the physicians at the disaster scene. The command center will direct ambulance transport of patients to appropriate hospital facilities. This center notifies the Dispatch Center of the destination of each ambulance, and in turn, the Dispatch center monitors the status of area hospital. It is essential that the Dispatch Center continually acquire information regarding hospital bed and resource availability and update and command center at least every 30 minutes during the evacuation phase of the disaster response. Each report from Dispatch Center should identify categorically the hospital's capabilities, particularly with respect to burn beds, trauma center beds, and intensive care beds. Using this data prevents overloading of trauma centers and local hospitals.

THE RESPONSE TO DISASTERS

Other
Center
Agencies

Resource
Regional
Dispatch
Hospitals

Hospitals/
Associate

POLICE

FIRE

Disaster
Communication
Matrix

Scene
Command
and
Communications
Centers

Ambulance Dispatch

Air Control/Resource

Rescue Triage Teams
DISASTER SITE

Disaster Scene

Figure 1

The site command post also coordinates communications with rescue triage teams assigned throughout the disaster area.

SECONDARY TRIAGE. The command center is a possible location for secondary triage, where victims receive interval therapeutics and prioritized transport to appropriate hospital resources. A staging area for ambulances and helicopters should be within close proximity. As indicated above, dispatch to hospital facilities ideally should occur from the command post, which is kept informed of the hospitals' status by the Dispatch Center.

MORGUE. A temporary morgue can be established near the command post, enabling both the police to maintain adequate security for the dead and their belongings, and the morgue teams to effect a relatively low-priority transport of bodies from the disaster site. If sufficient workers are available, the process of identifying the dead can begin at this time.

SUPPLY DEPOT. Ambulances returning from hospitals can deposit their supplies at the command post prior to departing with patients for the hospitals. The triage rescue teams, who are removing patients from the disaster site, then can bring supplies back to the patients left in that area. This allows orderly stocking of items, distribution of supplies to the triage rescue teams, and identification of needed items. (Fig. 2)

PHYSICIAN COMMAND. A physician experienced in emergency medicine should be present in the command center to work in concert with the designated fire or police official heading and coordinate the efforts of rescue triage teams, identify medical needs at the site, and oversee treatment and secondary triage.

Hospital

Hospital

Regional
Dispatch
Center

Ambulance

Patient
Pick-up

Figure 2

Organization at the scene of disaster.

Command Communications Center | Casualty Clearing Station | Supply Dump

Victims | Supplies

Rescue Triage Teams

Figure 3

RESCUE TRIAGE TEAMS

Emergency medical activity at the disaster scene is a team response which, under the direction of the disaster site physician, will identify the needs of the victims, provide primary assessment lifesaving therapeutics, and remove the victims from the site to the secondary triage area. (Fig. 3) Ideally, the team should consist of a paramedic, an EMT, a fire person for rescue and extrication, and a lay volunteer to help carry the stretcher. If available, a physician can be added to the team and should be added to the team if a patient is trapped or requires significant on-site medication. Communication among the team members is vital but is often difficult because the disaster site is hazardous and noisy. Each team should manage a specific limited physical area or pocket of the disaster. Thus more effectively responding to the injured. Therein, and then advising the command post of their readiness for future orders.

TRIAGE

The most crucial component of triage or sorting is identifying the severely injured patients, at risk of dying, whose lives could be saved by prompt treatment by capable facilities. Triage mechanisms must be simple and consistent (even when applied by different personnel) and have proven correlations with patient outcome for all types of trauma. Triage tags are rarely used in an actual disaster because they are not readily available; moreover, they require writing, which is frequently impossible at the site of primary triage and/or is inappropriately time-consuming. The rescue triage team leader will naturally respond to patients' needs in a prioritized manner, issuing appropriate orders and moving patients from the scene as rapidly as possible. Furthermore, the process of triage, which previously categorized patients into three or four triage, which previously categorized patients into three or four groups, based on urgency of needed treatment, is now more complex; this is reflected by the various echelons of prehospital care available and categorization of hospital facilities, particularly those with special care capabilities for trauma and burns. Finally, the use of triage tags discourage reevaluation of patient status at the disaster site.

One of the most critical functions performed by medical personnel is to classify or triage injured victims. The classification process is facilitated by use of the Revised Trauma Score, (RTS), physiological variables which allow for standardization of triage based on the central nervous, cardiovascular, and respiratory systems status.

The RTS is also used to prioritize transport to local hospitals for treatment. A prioritization scheme, similar to the following, may be utilized for transport.

This system is advantageous since it provides a standardized quantifiable numeric aid in triage, allowing for orderly victim assessment, despite a potentially chaotic environment. Some adjustment in the support priority scale may be necessary to address the availability of resources.

AIR COORDINATION

In certain disaster circumstances, helicopters have a role in both rescue and evacuation. A specific helicopter should be given command of their air space and should control the entrance and egress from this space by other helicopters. Helicopters can be based on distance from the disaster site and mobilized by the command helicopter for rescue or transport operations. The command helicopter communicates with the command post to ensure coordination of air evacuation with patient needs and land activities.

MEDIA

The press should not access the disaster site and instead, should receive information from a responsible authority through the command center. The press should be given details without speculation; unsubstantiated facts would not be relayed to the media. On the other hand, the microwave transmitters and mobile cameras of the press are an important resource that could improve disaster response. Responsible members of the media should work closely with disaster planners of the future to integrate the media's role in disaster activities.

STATE OR NATIONAL RESPONSE

In the event of a state or national disaster, it may be necessary to mobilize national resources, usually in the form of military or paramilitary personnel. The advantages of mobilizing these two bodies, in particular, are that they have their: 1) own resources; 2) communications systems; 3) high level of mobility; 4) mobile and fixed health care resources that can augment land, sea and air rescue and transport capability far in excess of local systems, and finally; 5) discipline in command/control procedures which are fundamental for a disaster response at any level.

REGIONAL DISASTER RESPONSE

The number of institutions and agencies involved in a regional response increase the likelihood of communications breakdown. This can be minimized by: (1) clearly defining the decision rules for a regional response; (2) identifying the mechanisms by which the response is to be coordinated; (3) maintaining the authority prerogatives of local jurisdiction; (4) identifying the command and control structure so it is easily recognized in the field and through the communications system; and (5) coordinating communications so that needs are consolidated intra-jurisdictionally before they are relayed to the regional disaster command structure.

SUBREGIONAL RESPONSE

A subregional response planning model requires all the components of the regional response. The actual process remains the same; however, the number and type of required resources should be somewhat less than required at the regional level, and slightly augmented from a local response.

LOCAL RESPONSE

The basic model, described herein, actually addresses response planning at the local level. Additional resources, as needed, augment the model when responding to higher level disasters.

TRANSPORTATION

To reiterate, dispatching ambulances, fire, and occasionally police vehicles should be coordinated through a Dispatch Center. This should minimize traffic jams and facilitate a more even distribution of transport vehicles.

The Command Physician should be responsible for establishing transport prioritization based upon the available personnel, supplies, transport vehicles and victim trauma scores. Although it is difficult to conduct time trials during a crisis, an attempt should be made to collect transit and routing data. This will be particularly useful during the post disaster evaluation of evacuation routes.

GEOGRAPHIC AND CULTURAL ADDRESS

Clearly, any disaster is complicated further by factors like inclement weather, terrain, and so forth. However, even greater complications arise when national boundaries overlap the disaster site. Language, equipment and even political incompatibility could hamper severely a disaster response especially if not previously addressed in the plan and if no practice drill was performed and evaluated.

POST-DISASTER EVALUATION

A retrospective review and evaluation of the disaster response is essential for future planning. Since most disaster plans are derived from the insights and anecdotes of those involved in previous disaster, it is important to analyze the elements of the response to any disaster. Once the facts have been collected, opinion can be incorporated as a step toward planning more effective responses in the future and disseminating any information not previously appreciated.

Decision trees are definitive, comprehensive, and explicit models of trauma management that can be used in the care of critically ill and injured patients during a mass casualty crisis. They are easily communicated verbally or in booklet form. Furthermore, they permit a core of experienced patient management specialists to effectively direct less experienced providers in various acute lifesaving clinical and surgical procedures.

Although the initial response in a disaster is correctly targeted toward the protection of life and limb and attaining and sustaining the physical well-being of those involved, psychiatric support is frequently required, both for the survivors of a disaster and for the personnel involved in the rescue and emergency medical responses. This latter group of individuals is frequently ignored; however, once the victims have been attended to, this group often merits attention because of a potentially negative psychological reaction to the experience.

CONCLUSION

Effective management of disasters historically has relied on the applicability of disaster plans, lessons learned from disaster drills, and coordination provided by Disaster and Emergency Preparedness Committees. Unfortunately, disaster plans are usually written once, updated periodically, and often do not take a realistic view of either the potential for certain types of disasters or the actual response of emergency personnel in those situations. While disaster drills test the entire response system, no simulation can approach the emergent nature of the tragic realism of an actual disaster. Although Disaster and Emergency Preparedness Committees draw together appropriate disaster-related agencies, they often fall prey to the political forces they are trying to coordinate and control.

Four components are essential to the successful handling of disaster. They are (1) medical command in the field, (2) a clear and visible hierarchy that delineates those in charge, (3) effective communication, and (4) appropriate and effective triage (sorting). The most frequent failure involves communications. The least developed area is that of patient triage. Satellites, cable TV, and media responsibility could improve the former; the latter must respond to tests of time and scenario. As the body of knowledge on disaster responses increases, all plans will be deficient in a particular disaster event, since requirement of flexibility does not allow it to dictate the minutia of reaction.

THE FRENCH ARMED SERVICES HEALTH DEPARTMENT: ITS ROLE FACING NATURAL DISASTERS

L.J. Courbil, M.D., Professor of Surgery
P. Chevalier, M.D., Anesthesiologist, Medical Advisor
J.L. Belard, M.D., M.Sc (Ergonomics and Human Ecology)

The Armed Services Health Department, Paris, France

INTRODUCTION

In France, the Armed Services Health Department plays a special and quite specific role in the way relief services are organized in daily emergencies and in major disasters.

As a joint agency of the Armed Services, its personnel may serve in the Army, the Air Force, the Navy or in the National Police Force, but they are also detached to other ministries. Therefore, while some personnel provide health support services for the Paris Fire Department, for the Marseille maritime firemen and civilian police forces, several hundreds military physicians take part in highway relief services, while five hundred military career physicians serve outside France under "Cooperation."

This availability and the variety of missions have been enshrined in the Health-Defense Agreements signed in 1982, one of the aspects of the coordination of civil and military resources when there are many victims, whether in times of peace or in times of war.

In the more distinct areas of disaster, there are a number of ways the Armed Services Health Department can play a role:

- on the regional or departmental (state) level, the Department may provide "mobile relief columns," whose personnel, posted near the emergency location, use their own evacuation resources and equipment and are prepositioned at certain regional sites and conditioned in the form of "disaster units." For example, under an ORSEC plan, the Prefect of a region may submit requests to the Ministry of Defense.

- on the national or international level, upon the request of a Ministry, such as Foreign Affairs, Cooperation, or the Ministry of the Interior, the Armed Services Health Department may provide large-scale relief by using autonomous and original units; i.e., l'Element Medical Militaire d'Intervention Rapide/EMMIR (the Military Medical Rapid Intervention Unit), the BIOFORCE and the Civilian Police Force Training Units.

Health and Medical Aspects of Disaster Preparedness
Edited by J.C. Duffy
Plenum Press, New York, 1990

DICA

DETATCHMENT D'INTERVENTION CATASTROPHE AEROMOBILE
AIRMOBILE DISASTER ASSISTANCE DETACHMENT

UISCs (Civilian Police Force Assistance Units) are military resources that are made available to the Ministry of the Interior to carry out tasks related to Civil Security in times of crisis.

The need to have an effective tool for major disasters led UISC/7, stationed in Brignoles, to develop a light detachment, adapted to risks, making it possible to provide a medical component on the front line and mobilize technical groups at the same time--all on both the national and international levels.

They have faced highly diverse situations, including earthquakes in El Asnam, Algeria (1980), Mezzo Giorno, Italy (1980), Mexico City (1985), Kalamta, Greece (1986); cyclones "Veena" in Tahiti (1983), "Kamisy" in Mayotte (1984); and attacks, such as the Drakkar post in Beirut, Lebanon, in 1983, where they assisted in the American zone as well, DICA has undergone changes several times as a result of lessons learned from experience.

A MULTIPURPOSE TOOL

DICA is fully autonomous for one week and can be ready to go within a maximum advance warning time of three hours, regardless of the duration and destination of the mission. This detachment can be deployed on the ground, even though it is mostly air-based. Its originality lies in its modular and threefold structure.

It includes 50 men, distributed as follows:

- an advance operational coordination detachment (DACO)
- a technical detachment (DT)

DACO is comprised of three sections:

- command and communications
- logistics
- medical

The medical section is comprised of three physicians and three nurses; its modular and threefold structure is the principle of its organization. It is modular because not all medical resources are required in all of the operations. It is threefold to make it possible for the medical team to act as a group or to be divided so that a physician and a nurse work with each of the three technical groups.

Therefore, the equipment includes three sets of portable medical kits, three sets of assistance kits for rough terrain, and a medical-surgical kit which includes three sets of seven field medical chests: surgical, asepticantiseptic-bandages-immobilization, circulatory, resuscitation, health assistance, pediatrics and tropical.

The BIOFORCE, created in 1983, is a very different unit intended to combat biological dangers such as epidemics. It was established by signing a memorandum of understanding that linked the Ministry of Defense, the Ministry of Cooperation, and the Pasteur and Merieux Institutes.

The physicians and nurses and the Armed Services Health Department, appointed in advance as in the case of EMMIR, are dispatched by military air transport. They use vaccines against cholera, yellow fever and cerebral-spinal meningitis provided by French industrial producers.

When an epidemic breaks out, a country asks the French public authorities for emergency assistance from the military BIOFORCE. Upon orders from the government, the Minister of Defense acts. In other words, he obtains the required vaccines from the Pasteur and Merieux Institutes, assembles the teams and the air resources and gives the BIOFORCE the order to depart right away.

Its missions have been accomplished over the last years using this arrangement:

In Madagascar (December 1984, May and April 1985), for an intensive vaccination campaign;

In Dkibouti (Christmas 1985, May 1986), with the same objectives;

In Guinea (April 1985) to eradicate a cerebral-spinal meningitis epidemic;

In Mali (1986), during a cholera epidemic.

EMMIR

I. MISSIONS AND OBJECTIVES

A. MISSIONS

Since its inception, EMMIR has undergone many changes and improvements and the new unit has become four times larger than the initial EMIR.

The various types of assistance it has effectively provided, and the assistance it is intended to provide, have demonstrated the absolute necessity of building a health unit with a sufficiently flexible structure to react quickly to a request for relief in any area and regardless of the type of disaster that justifies it.

Thus it became apparent that the unit could be called upon to take part in very different types of missions after natural or human disasters to care for the injured or the sick of both sexes, of any age, and do so using the most diverse specialties, such as surgery, medicine, pediatrics, epidemiology, etc.

Therefore, its field of activity has grown considerably. That is why EMMIR was designed to meet the following challenges:

- either a totally "surgical" mission - an emergency relief mission - such as that of the original EMIR. Under such circumstances, it could provide assistance:
    - o as it did in Jordan, when the civil war was winding down;
    - o or, for example, right after an earthquake;
- or a mission that involves medical services only;
    - o for refugees fleeing their countries for different reasons, such as war, epidemics, famine, etc.;

- or for a population group that is sometimes quite young and evacuated under the worst conditions; the best example was medical aid and treatment in Libreville for children brought from Biafra, hence, a significant pediatric component;

- or an epidemiological mission, because a Third World nation in difficulty could at any time request assistance in fighting an epidemic. The explosions of cholera in Chad and the Comores Islands, and smallpox in Somalia, only serve to substantiate this likelihood.

In fact, it is highly likely that in most cases EMMIR would be called upon to carry out combined missions:

- A combined medical and surgical mission:

  - this is the type of aid that is required just a few days after an earthquake occurs, such as the aid given to Peru, for example,

  - or aid that would be useful for displaced population groups, especially those in refugee camps.

- A combined medical-epidemiological mission:

  - attempting to prevent an epidemic from spreading,

  - and caring for population groups that have already been affected when the capacity of the health infrastructure that exists in the country has been more than saturated.

B. OBJECTIVES

The highly significant flexibility in use, which results from this adaptability, was one of the essential principles that was considered when the new version, EMMIR, was set up.

This unit's resources were altered as time went on. As its features changed, clear improvements were made in its capability of reacting to the following four requirements:

1. To meet all requests for relief quickly, wherever its assistance is justified, regardless of distance, altitude and climate. Hence, assistance everywhere.

2. To be assembled in less than 24 hours - both equipment and personnel. Hence, rapid intervention.

3. To have total autonomy in all areas, including supplies, communications, evacuations, etc. Hence, autonomous action.

4. To have a sufficiently flexible structure to take part in very different types of missions, such as a medical mission, surgical mission, combined mission, etc. Hence, adaptability of the unit.

A. Assistance Anywhere

Requests for assistance may come from very distant countries, such as Peru, Jordan, Nicaragua, Somalia, etc. The climates can vary greatly. Sometimes the unit may even be deployed at high altitudes. Anta in Peru is at an altitude of 2,600 meters. That is why requirements for deployment far from France have been studied--on the plain and in the mountains, in warm and cold climates--and related problems have been solved: distance, clothing, heating for tents.

1) Distance

Since 1970, the use of "C 160-Transall" military transport airplanes and their range has made it possible for EMMIR to reach the five continents quickly. For utilitarian or operational missions, these airplanes have already had to fly to nearly every corner of the world. The planes fly at 500 km an hour and have a range of up to 4,000 km and a load capacity of 6 to 10 tons, depending on the distance. Yet, even better performances are expected from the new series that has just been ordered.

One other essential quality of this airplane is its capability of landing on primitive grass landing strips less than 800 meters long. A striking demonstration of this occurred in Peru, where makeshift landing strips were often used. Therefore, thanks to this airplane's capabilities, it is likely that EMMIR will always be led to the heart of a disaster area on a relatively underdeveloped landing strip.

2) Clothing

Since they are called upon to serve in all places and in all climates, regardless of the weather, the personnel receives special clothing before they leave. The basic sets of clothing, as well as additional sets for "hot climates" and "cold climates," are in the inventory; and the personnel receive a down-lined jacket and a lined parka, as well as a bush hat and a light pair of shorts.

3) Heating

While waiting for heaters that can operate at any altitude to be installed, the tents are heated using different types of heaters (depending on whether they are used on the plain or in the mountains). It became apparent that highly sophisticated equipment worked very poorly at high altitudes, while the same equipment fared quite well at the seashore.

B. Speed of Intervention

Since its mission is to help the injured, it is rather obvious that relief must be provided on very short notice. The officers of the various operations that have already taken place unanimously agreed on this fact. To be operational within six hours was the essential criterion for the initial EMIR. In fact, it became apparent that for relief provided outside continental France, the advance notice had to be extended to 24 hours; thus, the orders to be ready within 24 hours were given and strict planning was set up to carry out the various duties for the personnel and equipment department.

Thus, deployment of the EMMIR mainly involves assembling for departure at a given plane the pre-selected personnel and equipment that will be required to carry out a specific relief mission.

Later we will see how the people are selected, how they reach their place of assembly, and how the equipment is taken to the very edge of the airfield from which the transport planes depart. Regardless, within a maximum of 24 hours, the personnel must reach the air terminal at the Air

Force Base in Orleans, the equipment must be loaded on the airplanes, and the various international administrative procedures must be completed for the entire EMMIR and related air detachments. Under such circumstances, at any minute and at any time of the year, the unit can be moved to the disaster area within 24 hours of receiving its orders.

So it happened when the unit left for Peru, and Jordan, and especially Nicaragua--when the unit was notified during the afternoon of December 24, and was assembled on Christmas night.

C. Autonomy In Action

In distress situations, the isolated rescue teams, and the units to an even greater extent, must not be a burden for the country that experiences the disaster, since all resources must be used to help the disaster victims. On the contrary, the relief units must work in a completely autonomous manner in a disaster area when its infrastructure is destroyed, when all sources of energy have been cut off, when communications have been severed, and when there is no transportation, medicine, food, and perhaps even no water. Therefore, the EMMIR must provide for:

- its own housing in tents,
- its own supplies; i.e.:
  - food,
  - potable water using reliable facilities,
  - medicine, using initial and maintenance lots that were brought along or shipped later.
- its own communications:
  - while using a team of specialists that has been made available, the need to have its own equipment became quite apparent during the initial missions.
- its own evacuations:
  - both from the site of the disaster back to EMMIR,
  - and from EMMIR to civilian hospitals, using its own self-propelled vehicles outfitted with stretchers, and its own air detachments, including airplanes and helicopters. Everything combined makes up the autonomous unit for humanitarian assistance from France.

D. Unit Adaptability

Since the EMMIR must:

- on one hand, be able to react on very short notice,

- and on the other hand, be able to accomplish different types of humanitarian missions,

- it had to be of an original design so that it did not waste time selecting and assembling the personnel and the equipment adapted to the specific mission at the time of departure for the disaster area.

That is why the unit was organized on a modular basis and formed from basic sections with their own personnel and equipment.

The organization is explained in the following.

II. ORGANIZATION

A. The EMMIR is a special kind of health unit.

In order to be able to respond quickly to the mission and to adapt to all circumstances, regardless of the distress situation, EMMIR has a modular design. Therefore, there are a number of autonomous basic sections, and each technical section is itself comprised of two identical teams. Moreover, EMMIR has different types of equipment, such as electrical generators, water purifying devices, etc..., and light vehicles.

The actual design of the unit makes it possible to easily combine one such section with another such section, as in a game of building blocks where the size and configuration of the building depends on the number and type of blocks that are used. However, each section, with its personnel and its highly specific and specialized equipment, forms a whole, even though the technical sections can be divided into two teams. This combination makes it possible to provide a different combination of resources for each request for assistance without any problems in order to adapt the unit to working conditions.

In one such case, for example, the EMMIR could be surgical, while in another, its mission will be of a medical nature. Elsewhere, its epidemiological variant will seem to be the most well adapted, and in other cases, the unit might deploy one or two sections of 50 beds.

In other words, the EMMIR offers the capability of providing 27 different combinations for a request, with a staff ranging from 24 to 78 persons and an overall equipment weight of 17 to 48 tons, including equipment not related to health.

These different capabilities, ranging from an exclusively medical to an exclusively surgical capability, with a medical-surgical capability in between, with or without a hospitalization component, make it possible to use the most logical relief unit possible, according to the known or presumed needs of the countries where disaster strikes.

Finally, each of these variants has a corresponding specific tonnage which is assessed immediately; this makes it possible to save an appreciable amount of time to prepare the flight plans for the transport airplanes and thus, to depart for the mission.

B. Structures

The EMMIR is comprised of six sections, each of which is distinct and independent from one another:

1. The "Command and Support" Section, including:

   a) "Headquarters" In charge of unit command, relations with the others and support functions.

   b) "General and Administrative Divisions," which have the following duties:

      Unit Management.

      Personnel management and management of equipment not related to health; supplies, food, transportation, etc...

Health Component Management:

Supervise patient arrivals, their civil status, accounting for money, health-related equipment, pharmacy, laundry, etc.

Attached to this section are:

o A "Transportation" team to drive and maintain service vehicles that have been brought along,

o A "Communications" team, if the operation takes place outside continental France, to provide various telecommunications.

2. "The Surgery Section"

This section includes two identical teams with the same equipment. It is supposed to classify the patients, bring them out of shock, bring them up to the conditions that will enable them to be evacuated, and even operate on them if necessary.

3. "The Medical Section"

This section is also comprised of two identical teams, at least one of which includes a pediatrician. Its mission is to see patients and take care of them and provide for hospitalization of patients and vaccinations.

4. The "Hospitalization" Section

This section is divided into two identical ones with 50 beds each. They are outfitted differently in order to care for either "medical" patients or "surgery" patients.

In its "medical" variant, it treats and houses patients either for a very short period or for while they wait for evacuation to hospitals.

In its "surgery" variant there is a team of surgeons. This enables them to accommodate people who have been operated on under the same conditions.

5. The "Laboratory" Section

Based on the same principle, there are two levels in this section:

- level one has basic supplies that enable it to do a minimum amount of laboratory testing,

- level two has more sophisticated supplies and a larger staff, as well as equipment that makes it possible to do special testing as dictated by different types of epidemics.

6. The "Air Convoy" Section

This section has two teams with the mission of providing medical supervision for injured people or patients while they are being evacuated by air.

III. OPERATIONS

A. Mobilization

1. Start-Up

a. General

Upon the request of a Ministry, such as Foreign Affairs, the Interior, or Public Health, and according to the specific case, the Government makes the decision to deploy the EMMIR and sees that the armed services notify the unit. Then air transport must take place no more than 24 hours after notification, assuming that flyover rights have been obtained. This implies:

- that the schedule of operations must be strictly observed so that the unit is ready within the appointed time frame;

- and that the time allotted for assembly is extremely short, since the people are scattered in different military hospitals throughout the country. Some are in Marseille, Bordeaux and Brest, which are far away.

This means that extremely explicit instructions have been given to the various authorities involved, both for moving the personnel to the departure point and for moving the equipment that belongs to the sections that take part in the mission.

b. Mobilization

In practice, unit mobilization involves the following three states:

(1) Early Warning

As soon as it is aware of a disaster, the Direction Centrale du Service de Sante/DCSSA (Central Health Department) collects as much information as possible about the disaster and the resources of the country affected, figures out the relief services that will be needed, and determines what resources can be sent.

As soon as it decides what type of EMMIR could be put into service for the situation, assuming that the Government would decide to take part in the relief effort, the DCSSA advises the regional departments from which personnel might be called.

Next these departments take all required steps to respond to the requests they might receive. However, it should be noted that it is not always possible to give the early warning and that the order to move may follow an announcement of the alert stage within 24 hours.

(2) Alert

Since the Government has made the Chiefs of Staff responsible for dealing with a possible deployment of the EMMIR, they must give the alert notice. The various Chiefs of Staff and the DCSSA, in their respective areas, transmit the orders that determine the "Health" resources, the transport resources, and the reinforcement resources (if need be) that have been chosen and are to be mobilized.

The alert means that the order to move may come within the next 24 hours.

(3) Order to Move

While the participation of the unit has been decided by the highest governmental authorities, the Chiefs of Staff order unit mobilization, define the resources, the means of transportation, and assign the order of take-offs. The Chiefs of Staffs that are involved react immediately, just like the DCSSA, and give the necessary orders.

c. Resource Assembly

(1) Personnel

Once the decision is made, the personnel assigned to the mission must react almost immediately. The specialists that serve at the Ecole Nationale des Sous-Officiers (National School for Non-Commissioned Officers) receive their own equipment and proceed to the military air station.

Those who come from the different units that belong to the three branches of the armed services and are scattered throughout the country immediately go to their place of assembly at Val-de-Garace. Those who are fartherest away use military or civilian air transportation. Then they are taken to the regional warehouse of the Health Department to receive their special packages and clothing. They are then taken by bus to the air force base from which they will depart.

(2) Equipment

At the same time, the sections, vehicles and equipment mobilized by the DCSSA are loaded on trucks according to the departure plan developed by the officers and taken to where they will receive their supplies at the military air base. The Air Force experts look after them and then they are boarded on cargo airplanes in accordance with the loading plan prepared by COTAM in cooperation with an officer of the Health Department appointed by DCSSA.

2. Transportation for the Unit

Transportation via highway or via railroad has not been used because the EMMIR was mainly designed for operation outside continental France. Most often, this requires rapid transportation via air. Nevertheless, there is no rule that prohibits all or a portion of the unit from being quickly dispatched to a disaster area in continental France as reinforcements under the ORSEC plan, for example. In such a case, transportation could be via:

- highway,
- railroad
- both highway and railroad, one after another.

However, the unit was especially designed for air transportation, and the military aircraft intended for this type of mission is primarily the NOR 2 501 transport aircraft, subsequently replaced with the C.160 Transall.

Transportation is implemented according to a plan prepared in advance by COTAM and is called "Operation Esculape." The plan determines the number of airplanes to be deployed according to the distance to be traveled, possible stops along the way, and the tonnage.

3. Deployment

a.) Procedures

Upon arrival in the country that requested the international assistance, the Chief Physician of the unit:

- introduces himself to the authorities that greet him and to the French representatives posted in the country,

- identifies the technical capabilities and working conditions of the EMMIR,

- obtains the orders concerning his role in the overall relief scheme from the accredited officials and is given a specific mission,

- if possible, inspects the site where the EMMIR will be located before the unit goes there.

At the disaster area, while the unit is on its way, the Chief Physician establishes personal communications with the different authorities already at work, including the military, rescue teams, etc., and prepares for his hospital's deployment.

b. Deployment

(1) Terrain Features

Depending upon the circumstances, all or a portion of the EMMIR may be deployed:

- either in quarters in existing buildings, at the close of a civil war, for example,

- or in bivouac in tents, in a totally devastated area, where there is an earthquake, for example.

Both of these procedures obviously have advantages and disadvantages, but regardless of the type of deployment, there must be:

- enough room for all of the unit,
- the ability to set up a landing area for helicopters,
- proper water supply to the extent possible,
- ease of automobile traffic, if possible.

Especially when the disaster area is vast, the unit must be located as close to a landing strip as possible, even if it is a grass landing strip, so that the C.160 Transalls can use it, because they will play an essential role in evacuating injured people that have been treated and in supporting the unit.

(2) Signage

The unit is identified both on the ground and in the air by the emblems of the Red Cross. The national flag may fly next to that of the nation that is receiving the assistance as long as approval has been obtained from the authorities in charge.

(3) Housing in Tents

This is the only type of housing planned. However, it is important to note that each type of deployment has its own number of corresponding tents that are to be brought along, according to the number of sections that comprise the mission.

- Number of Tents

The smallest unit, with only one medical team, should bring along two tents that will be reserved for the technical divisions and two tents for the general divisions, for a total of four tents. On the other hand, a fully deployed unit would have 31 standard tents and 5 cross configuration tents distributed as follows:

	Cross Configuration Tents	Standard Tents: Operational Tents	Standard Tents: Hospital Tents	Standard Tents: Service Tents
Command...				5: 1 kitchen 1 cafeteria 1 headquarters 1 housing 1 communications (technical & housing)
Surgery...	2	2	5	1 housing
Medicine...	1		4	1 housing
Hospitalization	2		10	2: 1 housing 1 storage
Laboratory...				1 housing & technical
	5	2	19	10
TOTAL	5		31	

- Area required for installation
  - minimum for 4 tents........................ 600 m^2
  - for the entire unit........................ 10,000 m^2

- Tent features:

  Tents used are 1960 type Health Department tents with metal frames. They are easy to put up and do not require a central pole. The tents measure 8 m x 5.4 m; the height in the middle is 2.7 m at the peak, and the ground area is 43.2.m^2. Each tent can accommodate 10 to 12 cots. All the tents look alike on the outside. However, the "hospitalization" tents and the "operating" tents are different from the "service" tents because there is an added special interior awning and a removable ground rug. Moreover, some tents may be divided into compartments using fabric for separation that forms a "wall." The radiology, laboratory and pharmacy tent has a special awning that makes it possible to obtain a number of "rooms," including a darkroom.

- Time required for deployment:

  The amount of time required for deployment on appropriate and cleared land is as follows:

surgery tent..............	4 hours
medicine tent.............	1.5 hours
hospitalization tent......	2.5 hours
command tent..............	3 hours
lab tent..................	1 hour
for the entire unit.......	15 hours

Technical tents and a portion of the hospitalization tents are put up on a priority basis so that they can be opened for admissions as early as possible. In theory, they open at hour # 3 for surgery and hour # 6 for hospitalization. Obviously, these minimum times are only for a preliminary installation of the tents and preparation of first aid equipment.

In reality, available personnel are used to finish the installation and prepare the entire unit over several days. They dig the ditches around the tents, install the x-ray and laboratory machinery, arrange the pharmacy, set up the kitchens, etc...

4. Health Supplies

Considering the significant requirement for potable water, water supply must be as effortless as possible. The ideal situation would be to set up camp around a water hole.

The EMMIR arrives on the scene with health supplies that will enable it to work from one to four weeks, depending upon the quality of the maintenance kits that were brought along at departure time.

Later, an air shipment of one or more kits, taking into account the duration of the stay, may be requested from France, if the unit has not been able to replenish its supply of depleted items locally.

Finally, special requests may be made to replenish first aid equipment before it is depleted. All such requests are made directly to France through the unit's "communications" resources.

5. Communications

The EMMIR communicates with the outside mainly as follows:

- by wire, with the different agencies of the host country and other relief units, if the local authorities took part in installation,

- by radio, in which case the communications section has the following mission:

  o to communicate:

  - with the French Embassy in order to facilitate communication with the various agencies of the country in which the disaster occurred and solve the many problems that arise when such a unit goes into action in a foreign country and in a disaster environment,

  - with France, whatever the distances, in order to tell of the unit's needs, such as food, medicine, spare parts, etc..., and to give periodic news of the personnel.

  o to monitor air resources during their air missions:

  - first, with the helicopters that remain based with the EMMIR, and which are used occasionally under rather difficult circumstances in the work area for which they were made responsible,

  - and additionally, the transport airplanes which are in communication with the host base to which they have been assigned.

Contacts are made with the different correspondents one or more times each day, according to:

- orders from the Chiefs of Staff of the Armed Forces

- and the duty schedules with the different authorities to be contacted.

IV. AN EXAMPLE

PERU - June 14 - July 6, 1970

On May 31, 1970, a very powerful earth tremor hit an entire region of Peru. The epicenter was in the ocean, a few kilometers from Chimbote, Peru's major port, and 400 km north of Lima, on the Pacific Coast. The seismographs recorded a reading of 7.75 on the Richter scale. Even in Lima, despite the distance, the shock was felt and cracked walls.

The disaster was wide in scope. About 128,000 km^2, or one-fourth of the country, was devastated, and of that, over 80,000 km^2 were 100% devastated. Two hundred and fifty cities and towns were left in ruins and reduced to rubbish. Two hundred thousand houses were destroyed.

Since the event occurred in one of the most densely populated areas of Peru, there were 3,470,000 people involved and 800,000 of them were totally affected by the disaster and lost everything. There were many injured - over 140,000 - with about 3,000 seriously injured, and the number of dead rose above 65,000.

A. Organization of Relief Efforts

It took the Peruvian Government several days to realize how serious the disaster was because telephone communications were totally cut off. Bridges, roads and railroads in one entire province were destroyed. Moreover, the province is mountainous and covers the two Cordilleras.

The disappearance of Yungay, a vacation resort with 25,000 inhabitants, was only discovered one week later. Much later, it was discovered that a passenger train was lost in a tunnel under the del Pato Canyon.

However, the relief services were organizing. A "Junta de Assistencia Nacional" coordinated the resources. The Army brought together men and equipment. Soon, the parachutists would jump to repair small landing strips to make it possible for small aircraft to land.

Solidarity was quick to transcend the borders! The neighboring countries of South American and Central America dispatched blankets, tents and food. Voluntary rescue teams came from all over the world.

Finally, realizing the scope of the disaster, Peru made an appeal on June 10 for international solidarity, and it was heard throughout the world. The United States had its aircraft carrier, the Guam, change course on its way back from Vietnam. The Brazilians dispatched a number of helicopters and the Canadians sent several "Caribous," cargo airplanes that can land on makeshift landing strips. West Germany opened a rural hospital and France also decided to provide assistance.

B. The Relief Mission: Start-Up

In Paris, on June 10, the Cabinet decided to answer the appeal it had just received from the government.

The Minister of Defense offered to send a military medical assistance mission and the EMMIR was put on alert the same day with related detachments: airplanes and helicopters.

1. Mission Composition

The Armed Services Chiefs of Staff ordered that the following three components be set up:

a. The Air Transport Group:

Four C.160 "Transall" cargo planes were to fly the EMMIR and three helicopters. Once that was completed, two aircraft stayed at the base to support the unit while the other two returned to France 48 hours later. The two aircraft that stayed were to bring the personnel back. The equipment would return by ship. However, the two aircraft that were scheduled to return stayed at the base for 10 days to carry out the many missions that awaited them before they returned to the base from which they departed.

The Group included 32 crew members, 7 ground staff and 4 officers in charge of the aircraft, for a total of 43 persons. Two thousand one hundred kg of technical equipment were brought in the aircraft bays. The crews were highly experienced and perfectly trained to use the makeshift landing strips.

b. Helicopter detachment:

The Army's Light Aviation Group, whose home base is Pau, at the foot of the Pyrenees, supplied a detachment of three Alouette III's. There were 12 staff people, 6 pilots with experience flying in mountainous areas, a ground officer and five mechanics who were in charge of 800 kg of technical equipment. These aircraft can carry either three seated passengers or 300 kg of freight.

c. The EMMIR

Twenty-eight people comprised the EMMIR: 12 physicians, 1 manager, 6 noncommissioned officers and 9 privates. But locally, the four officers in charge of the aircraft asked to serve in the hospital, thereby bringing the total number to 32.

Because the earthquake occurred on May 31, and because the equipment was used so late, a number of additional lots of medicine were provided in order to make both medical activity and surgery possible over four weeks. Additional maintenance supplies, medical field chests from abroad, free medical assistance, additional technical supplies and war rations were added to the initial supplies, thereby raising the tonnage to 20 tons.

2. Mission Installation

On June 11 the personnel assembled in Orleans and waited for the order to take off - it was finally given on June 12. Four Transall airplanes left the base one after another. Two of them landed in Pau to pick up the helicopters. On June 14, after stops in Cape Verde, Recife and Manaus, the airplanes arrived in Lima.

On June 15 there was a meeting to explain to the Peruvian authorities that the French rescue mission was to be an effective whole with real operational capabilities as long as it was not split apart. The Peruvians agreed to let the unit remain intact and they assigned it a series of tasks.

Immediately, the officers of the three detachments went to the heart of the disaster area to inspect the host area. It was located at the center of a heavily affected geographical area, where communications had not yet been restored with Lima or with Chimbote on the coast. The paratroopers found a grass landing strip which was partially obstructed by earth that had caved in. Thus, the Transalls would be able to land and the EMMIR and the Alouettes would be able to settle in close to the strip.

Three hundred fifty km northwest of Lima, halfway between Huallanca to the North, and Recuay to the South, right in the middle of the disaster, the makeshift landing strip at Anta was set up for light airplanes bringing tourists who were going to Yungay to rest and skiers tempted by the great Huascaran (6,787 m), the second highest peak in South America.

The center of the relief effort, where the light airplanes and helicopters brought in the equipment and the rescue teams, came to be located in Callejon de Huaylas, a valley at an altitude of 2,600m, suspended between Black Cordillera and White Cordillera, at the center of what the reporters would come to call "Death Valley." The Peruvian Army set up its command post and coordination post there. The Brazilians based their "Iroquois" helicopters there.

Until that point, the landing strip had only been used by Peruvian, Brazilian and Venezuelan C47s, Argentine Fikkers and Canadian Caribous. In terms of "Health," a Peruvian medical unit with limited resources located there, and volunteer physicians and nurses from the United States, Canada and Cuba came to offer their services.

On June 16, the planned movement took place without a hitch and the four Transalls landed. Minutes later, an "Alouette III" brought in a German skier in difficulty. He was trapped for 10 days on the slopes of Huascaran at an altitude of 4,200 meters; this also demonstrated the operational capabilities of these aircraft and their crews.

The EMMIR located beyond the overburdened area of the parking lots and their immediate surroundings, overrun with lines of refugees awaiting their turn to board, with peasants used to unload airplanes and Peruvian soldiers on duty on the area. The helicopters stayed in the middle and the airplanes returned to Lima as the first planes of an air bridge that would be flown on a daily basis.

After nearly thirty hours of flight, the altitude and the hot sun (35° C in the shade), everyone watched his efficiency drop.

Nevertheless, on June 17, the hospital was fully ready and set up in the shape of an "X" around a cross configuration tent; the first surgical operation was able to take place the same day early in the evening. Two tents with 12 examining tables were reserved for the reception area and classifying the injured. The operation section and five resuscitation beds were located in the two other tents. Hospitalization had 18 beds in two tents.

The EMMIR personnel was housed in two tents outfitted with 30 stretchers, while ALAT personnel and the air strip officers occupied two small camping tents on loan from the local authorities.

Other similar tents made it possible to set up medical and surgical consultation centers, storage areas, cafeterias, kitchens, etc., in the coming days.

Similarly, 30 metal beds, complete with linens, quickly replaced the unit's cots, which were given to personnel who only had stretchers issued to them until that point.

Finally, the workers found among the refugees quickly made improvements in the area surrounding the hospital and its appearance from the outside, which included alleys with old fences, primitive shelters to protect the cafeterias, electrical generators, the shower, etc... From that point on, the French camp in overall terms looked quite presentable and just as nice as that of the different units located in Anta.

C. Mission Activity

1. Mission Identification

Upon the request of the two officers of the "medical" and "helicopters" detachments, the Commander of the disaster area put the French in charge of an area of about 100 km long and 30 km wide. Anta was located in the middle and the area was centered on the Rio Santa, which spans the Callejon de Huaylas from east to west.

The area could be identified using several points:

- average altitude, 2,700m, between 4,870 m in the west and 6,800 m in the east, where the snows begin,

- the most densely populated area of Peru, with a few towns from 10,000 to 25,000 inhabitants, and villages located at an altitude of up to 4,500 m,

- an area heavily affected by the disaster, with houses destroyed or buried by alluvial soil which came down from the mountains; also, diminished communications to the villages located at high altitudes and severed communications at many points in the valley.

2. EMMIR Activity

Once the hospital opened and the first missions were accomplished in the surrounding villages, the EMMIR began its essential mission as follows:

- it systematically identified and injured people in the villages scattered over the mountain and took them to the hospital,

- it provided surgical treatment for the injured people that were found, and medical treatment as well, owing to the living conditions of the people,

- in the villages they visited they collected information on the magnitude of the injuries, the disaster victims and damages, all upon the request of the authorities and the needs that resulted from their findings.

However, once the initial visits to the villages began, a fourth mission turned out to be essential: to comfort the Indian groups who were still traumatized, fatalistic by nature and still affected by a catastrophe which renders mankind powerless.

a. Activities in the villages:

Each morning, two "Alouette III's" flew in formation as a security precaution and, in an isolated village affected by the disaster, on the slopes of the Cordilleras surrounding the valley, dropped off two medical teams, comprised of one physician and a nurse or medical officer, for a stay that could be long or short, depending upon the size of the population, but never longer than one day.

Once the team met the local authorities they were taken to the injured and the ill, where they consulted with them, provided first aid, made bandages, decided if it was necessary to evacuate, collected any information on the disaster, and prepared a needs statement for the authorities as well as requests for emergency relief to which the helicopters would respond that day or the next. It should be mentioned that of 61 villages visited, 57 were 100% destroyed!

During that time, the helicopters made countless round trips to bring those people who were evacuated to the hospital and bring in food, equipment, and especially blankets. Regardless, the hospitality was warm because in most cases no one had yet visited the villages, and no assistance was provided. The medical teams also informed the local people of the extent of the national disaster.

However, these population groups were quite exhausted. Anguish and fear were still visible on everyone's face, caused by the earthquake and prolonged by small but frequent aftershocks. Furthermore, many families preferred to continue living in nothing more than huts that were built after the earthquake. Such shelters were almost worthless, because even though the thermometer climbed to nearly 60° C during the day, it fell to minus 10° C during the night in villages located at high altitudes.

However, the teams were received with great sympathy, and from their voyages, they told of heartbreaking scenes. The people, who had been isolated since the disaster, found much comfort, both physical and moral, from those who rescued them, which counteracted their natural fatalism.

At the end of the day, the two officers of the Health and Helicopters detachment reported to the Peruvian General, who was in charge of the area, on requests made by the disaster victims. They prepared for the work to be done the next day by choosing the villages to be visited.

b. Hospital activity:

Located at the heart of the disaster area, and right next to the relief coordination center, the hospital would play the role of an area hospital. After the small Peruvian hospital was dismantled and evacuated on June 19, this hospital was the only properly equipped one in the area. It carried out two types of activities:

- consultations,
- hospitalizations.

(1) Consultations:

Consultations were available to people who lived close to the hospital during the first days; then, as people found out where it was, they came from much farther away. Actually, there were few operations performed that were related to the earthquake, which had occurred three weeks earlier. Rather, there were medical consultations related to living conditions, poor housing and food. The pathology was similar in every detail to that treated by the traveling teams.

(2) Hospitalizations:

The few injured people found in the villages were taken to the hospital if necessary, sometimes on stretchers or on horseback from the nearby villages, but mostly by either French or foreign helicopters.

The "Alouettes" were not the only ones to work for the hospital. The Brazilians, with their "Iroquois," and even the Americans brought the injured people they found in their work areas to the EMMIR. Those who were only slightly injured were kept a few days if necessary. The more severe cases received the necessary primary care and were evacuated as quickly as possible to hospitals in Lima.

The hospital had only 30 beds. There were also camping tents set up to receive the most benign cases for treatment. Every day, a Transall ambulance airplane made it possible to carry out secondary sanitary evacuations under the best circumstances. However, the hospital soon opened to medical cases and they quickly outnumbered surgical cases. Thus, the hospital was operating at capacity.

Nevertheless, the occupancy rate never exceeded 50%, thanks to air evacuations. In fact, the rate was intentionally maintained at 50% in order to make it possible to accommodate unanticipated overcrowding, due either to heavier arrivals of the ill or the injured, or to a temporary closing of the landing strip due to weather.

3. Air Detachment Activity

a. Helicopters:

Their activity was:

- first and foremost in support of the medical teams,
- but also in support of the Peruvian authorities.

In the first case, they hauled the teams to the villages located at high altitudes and brought back the injured and the ill to the hospital.

In the second case, they brought engineering technicians to the site, mostly so that they could inspect the many lakes that had been created with artificial dams that could break. They also brought soldiers and officials and of course, equipment, blankets and food, to the most severely affected victims, according to the orders of the relief coordination command post.

b. C.160 Transalls

They provided:

- veritable air bridge between Lima, their home base, and Anta,
- air transportation upon request.

The air bridge between Lima and Anta made it possible to do the following on a daily basis:

- to evacuate the injured and haul refugees on the one hand,
- and on the other hand, to bring supplies to the hospital, move rescue teams, military units and equipment that were to be given to the disaster victims.

Air transportation between Lima and other landing strips was provided for different types of equipment, such as bulldozers, compressors, etc., when so requested by the Peruvian authorities.

D. End of Mission and Return

The number of injured people treated decreased slowly but surely. The major work was over. The roads to Lima were reopened. The disaster area was inspected and the urgent needs were met. Rescue activities declined regularly and the foreign rescue teams, whether isolated or in formation on the Guam, the U.S. aircraft carrier, or Canadian Caribous, on American C.130's, or on Brazilian helicopters, returned to their countries on June 26.

Following the advice of the chief of mission, the French Ambassador proposed that all activity cease on July 6. While the first half of the personnel were taking their turn enjoying two days of relaxation in Cuzco and in Macchu-Pichu, the Inca capital, the other half were dismantling the hospital and repacking the equipment for the return.

On July 7, the medicine and the consumables, such as bandages, blankets, etc., were handed over to the Peruvian authorities. The equipment was sent back to France via ship and the personnel returned on board the Transall airplanes.

E. Mission Results

The mission was operational for 19 days, from June 17 to July 6, 1970.

The results are as follows:

1. Activity of the traveling teams;

- 44 teams deployed,
- 61 villages visited,
- 2,143 consultations,
- 50 primary evacuations.

2. Hospital activity:

- 1,229 medical consultations,
- 177 surgical consultations,
- 44 operations (9 under general anesthesia),
- 2 deaths (2 children with 100% burns).

3. Air resources:

- 58 primary evacuations via helicopter,
- 66 secondary evacuations via Transalls.

V. CONCLUSIONS ON EMMIR OPERATIONS

EMMIR's experiences made a considerable contribution to the Armed Services Health Department. In particular, they made the following possible:

- for personnel, to have men and women who were constantly trained and motivated for group emergency situations

- for equipment, to constantly test new equipment and seek solutions for the many problems that arise in critical situations of resuscitation (for example, blood transfusions or supply of oxygen)
- for rules, to understand the priority requirements for classifying patients, which is the basis of efficient and cost-effective medical activity.

Thus, a simple series of categories was adopted, which makes a distinction between:

- ABSOLUTE emergencies in which the issue is vital prognosis

- and RELATIVE emergencies in which treatment may be postponed without any vital risks, but simply at the expense of a subsequent functional prognosis.

On the other hand, among the absolute emergencies, although most require surgery as early as possible, some operations are not necessarily done by a surgeon.

Thus, POTENTIAL emergencies, frequent in disaster situations when there area areas that are buried, are mainly the responsibility of the supervision of a therapist; IRREVERSIBLE emergencies, due to the seriousness of their condition and minimal chances of survival, must wait for others to be treated who have better chances in situations where equipment shortages are typical of disasters.

CONCLUSIONS

The Armed Services Health Department derived different benefits from these missions:

1) Its reputation in the country improved and the concept of an integrated Army and Navy was appreciated by all.

2) Its personnel, whose motivation and willingness to serve were constantly being tested, demonstrated their determination through their prolonged volunteerism and thus are always prepared for emergency situations.

3) The new equipment is constantly under experimentation in critical situations.

4) The principles of medicine in disasters become more solid and improve constantly. The Armed Services Health Department published these principles recently in "Medicine en situation de catastrophe - S.S.A.," Masson Publishers, Paris, 1987. Moreover, its specialists teach in several medical schools as part of a university degree called "medicine for disasters."

VA HEALTH CARE SYSTEM EXPERIENCE WITH NATURAL DISASTERS

Mark W. Wolcott, M.D.

Assistant Chief Medical Director
U.S. Veterans Administration
for Clinical Affairs
Washington, D.C.

INTRODUCTION

At 7:42 a.m., on October 1st, 1987, an earthquake measuring 6.1 on the Richter scale struck the Los Angeles area.

Effects of the earthquake were felt as far south as San Diego and as far north as San Luis Obispo.

While 16 aftershocks measuring two or three on the Richter scale continued to rock the metropolitan area, a major mobilization of emergency teams took place and as casualty and damage reports came in, two things became clear.

First, although damage was fairly widespread, the ultimate severity in terms of casualties and property damage was relatively minor compared with the consequences of other major seismic events.

Second, the response by disaster emergency forces was swift, well-organized, and comprehensive.

With a powerful array of emergency medical teams, utility damage control units and safety and public health officials assembled in a remarkably short period of time.

Both of the facts reflect, to a considerable degree, preparations by the engineering and medical communities.

This is not surprising; there is extensive and widely reported scientific knowledge about the long-term potential of coastal California's San Andreas fault system to produce a major seismic event in the next 30 years.

In fact, in reporting about this latest disaster, Los Angeles area news media referred to the likelihood of a major earthquake as part of the lore and life style of living in Southern California.

But one segment of the community - those who work in the Veteran's Administration (VA) Health Care System - had particularly ominous feelings when this earthquake occurred. Their collective memory was focused on another date: February 9, 1971.

Health and Medical Aspects of Disaster Preparedness
Edited by J.C. Duffy
Plenum Press, New York, 1990

At just after 6:00 a.m., that Tuesday morning, an earthquake measuring 6.5 on the Richter scale struck near the same area of Los Angeles.

That time, it was devastating, killing 62 people, injuring hundreds and causing damage estimated at more than one billion dollars.

The epicenter was in the San Fernando valley, and the VA's 426-bed General Medical and Surgical Hospital in that area was at "ground zero."

Two bed buildings in the center of the VA Hospital complex collapsed, killing thirty-eight patients and ten employees.

Water, telephone, and electrical services were cut over a wide area, and residents were evacuated for days until structural studies could determine the safety of surviving structures.

Eventually, the San Fernando VA Medical Center had to be closed and completely demolished.

Background

Comprehensive comparisons of the 1971 and 1987 earthquakes in Los Angeles have not been completed. So the degree to which sounder construction and variance in seismic severity influenced outcomes of these two events cannot yet be demonstrated.

Nevertheless, it's apparent that a number of advances in the area of disaster response have occurred in the intervening years.

For example, emergency medicine is now a recognized medical specialty, clinical support services have advanced, and emergency communications systems have been revolutionized.

This movement has been national in scope, facilitated through the Emergency Medical Services Systems Act of 1973, and subsequent amending legislation.

But the general advance of medical science and federal guidance alone do not explain the difference in responses between the two California earthquakes.

It's quite clear that local planning was responsible for much of the progress, reflecting that special experience from the past event contributed to improved performance in the second.

This observation underscores two rather basic questions:

First: Do those of us who are concerned, not with emergency planning, but with operational, clinical medicine, take disaster planning seriously enough in between earthquakes?

Second: Should we all be more interested in the lessons from past natural disasters because of the way they might contribute to better planning for the future?

The answer to the first question is powerfully demonstrated by the rather startling statistics on the prevalence of natural disasters.

In an average year, about five hurricanes will "come ashore" in the continental United States, and some 900 tornadoes will touch down.

Even more remarkable, the National Earthquake Information Center predicts 1200 to 1500 earthquakes of varying magnitudes in the U.S.

The National Association of Fire Prevention predicts an astonishing 2.3 million fires will take place in this country.

To the extent that medical facilities traditionally plan a pivotal role in responding to emergencies, it's obvious that this large number of disasters will involve many health care professionals in a substantial way.

Moreover, juxtaposing this great prevalence of natural disasters with the wide dispersion of 6,850 hospitals in America...makes it apparent that many medical facilities themselves will be -- like our San Fernando VA Hospital -- the site of a disaster.

In this context, the VA's distinction as the Nation's largest health care system is not so positive. Our 172 medical centers and dozens of smaller, stand-along facilities do comprise more "targets" than any other single system; and in the 41-year history of the VA's department of medicine and surgery, we've had experience commensurate with those opportunities.

A salient point in this history is that the ability of individual facilities within our system to respond to medical emergencies has varied tremendously depending upon the specific mission of that facility. Even today, there is a substantial spectrum of capabilities. At one end, typically at our university affiliated centers, we have leading edge trauma centers...such as that at our Albuquerque shared facility with the Air Force...with multidisciplinary teams and specialized surgical suites, backup generation and emergency medical gas supplies sustaining full patient monitoring and life support equipment.

At the other extreme, we have some smaller facilities which can marshall only very basic, primary services.

Statement of Purpose

Nevertheless, many elements of facility response to disasters are common to all our locations. With a view that past experience is of value in considering the way disaster planning has progressed, we set about making a brief review of VA's experience with natural disasters.

Methodology

As I will further detail in a moment, developing and managing individual disaster response programs is largely decentralized in the VA system. For this reason, and since policy on reporting details about natural disaster has varied substantially over the years, there is no single, comprehensive repository of data concerning natural disasters in the VA.

Our review, therefore, entailed not only a search for records in various offices of our headquarters in Washington, D.C., but a system-wide request for information about individual facility experience with natural disasters.

Interestingly, we found that one of the most extensive bodies of records exists within our medical facility construction program. It would appear that, in some cases, our facilities have provided rather sketchy documentation of disasters to operational offices, but they've been quite cooperative in providing extensive detail to those responsible for rebuilding and reequipping their physical plants.

In any case, we determined that a strict, data-oriented approach was not possible because comprehensive details are not available on all disasters.

We therefore reviewed the data available in a somewhat anecdotal fashion, attempting to select representative cases of response to various categories of natural disasters.

As part of this process, we compared VA actions with some general references on emergency medical service systems, Triage, and other relevant activities in disaster circumstances. For example, we considered initial emergency medical actions performed during disaster in the context of those prescribed in the reference "Triage" by Rund and Rausch. We evaluated the process of transferring patients to external emergency trauma services based on definitions suggested in the AHA's text, "The Hospital's Role in Emergency Medical Services Systems."

We then considered the extent to which the VA experiences have contributed to current disaster response plans in place in VA facilities.

Mortality/Morbidity

In every natural disaster involving VA facilities, reports were made, and inquiries conducted into, instances of patient death. I will reference these in a moment as I discuss individual cases.

Morbidity -- as is always the case -- was far more difficult to assess. Data collected in virtually all instances of natural disaster include physical injuries sustained, but psychological effects were noted in only a few instances.

Based on the limited number of observations which were adequately recorded, it is accurate to say that some adverse effects occurred in every instance of disaster, primarily because of the interruption of treatment programs.

Typical effects noted included delays in appropriate therapy, medication errors, and duplication of diagnostic procedures.

Specific Review of Experiences

For purposes of this review, we divided our experiences with natural disasters into six categories: Fires, floods, hurricanes, tornadoes, "human inspired events," and earthquakes.

1. Togus Fire

The realm of Veterans Health Care had its first experience with natural disaster not only before establishment of VA's Department of Medicine and Surgery in 1946, but before veterans programs were consolidated into the Veterans Administration in 1930.

This initial calamity took place only two years after the end of the Civil War, at a facility known as the National Home for Disabled Volunteer Soldiers, in Togus, Maine.

At half past nine in the evening of January 7th, 1868, the home's heating system started a fire which ultimately destroyed the main building. At the time, the home housed 270 disabled veterans, 31 of whom were acutely ill.

The small staff, aided by the more able-bodied veteran patients, evacuated the facility which burned to the ground.

The Commandant of the home was not in attendance at the time, and command of the emergency fell to the chief surgeon. This physician's major problem was the severe cold -- and the fact that there was no shelter.

Messengers were sent to nearby Augusta, Maine, for assistance, but, meanwhile the veterans themselves took action against the elements. In the surgeon's stores, which survived the fire, was a barrel of whiskey for the usual medicinal purposes. The veterans appropriated it to fight off the freezing weather.

The Surgeon duly reported this development, and described the condition of his patients--and I quote: "The soldiers drank to such an extent that they became beastly drunk, and disgusting scenes of disorder and violence ensued."

Rescue teams finally arrived, and all of the patients were taken to Augusta, where they were quartered in private homes and the town hall. One veteran died from exposure.

In the best tradition of analyzing a disaster to improve future readiness, an inquiry was conducted into the incident, resulting in two recommendations:

- First, fire resistant materials should be used in rebuilding the home;

- Second, a class in deportment should be taught to the veteran patients.

2. New Orleans Fire

There have been more serious examples of fire disaster in our system, and a case in point took place at the New Orleans VA Medical Center.

This incident involved one of the greatest fire dangers to the modern hospital.

We've seen that, while fire cannot sweep through today's structures as rapidly as it did through older, wooden buildings, dense smoke from burning modern materials can spread through a modern hospital even more rapidly than in older buildings, because of today's extensive air duct systems.

Our problem in new Orleans began during construction on a clinical addition, when a contractor's cutting torch ignited materials in a storage room.

A number of the hospital's sprinkler and alarm systems were temporarily out of service during the construction, so the fire burned for nearly one and a half hours before being extinguished. Heavy smoke spread through several areas of the hospital.

The brighter side of this picture was that, in the absence of the facility's automatic fire safety systems, the human response was excellent.

Once the fire was discovered, prompt and efficient action was taken to rescue endangered individuals, to contact fire fighters, and to protect patients from possible injury.

The clinical staff performed with great presence of mind and professionalism during this emergency. This was responsible for the fact that there was no loss of life due to the fire.

The influx of smoke through the ventilation system made it necessary to evacuate several wards. Patients were moved by staff and volunteers to the VA's outpatient clinic in an adjoining building.

Triage was performed in the clinic admitting area by a team of VA residents and nurses.

A small number of acutely ill patients were transferred to two community hospitals; others were made comfortable in the clinic area while fans cleared the air in the bed building.

The medical intensive care unit had to be evacuated, and six acutely ill patients were transferred by special ambulance to the ICU of a nearby community hospital.

Three patients and seven staff members sustained minor injuries, either sprains or bruises incurred in the evacuation.

Smoke and water damage was fairly extensive. The greatest single loss involved monitoring equipment in the MICU, which was completely destroyed. Total cost of the incident was $594,000.

Lessons from the experience included:

- o That great care must be taken whenever safety systems are disabled during construction.

- o There must be plans to augment the standard telephone service for emergency communications. This observation is a common thread running through modern VA experience with disasters.

A natural reaction is to pick up the telephone to ask what's going on, and this obviously overloads the standard means of communicating emergency information.

An important, underscored note on VA Disaster Plans today is the reminder -- on every page -- to use telephones only for official emergency business.

3. Cheyenne Flood

The opposite end of the spectrum from fire presents different considerations, but provides not less challenge for disaster planning.

One of our most notable flood experiences took place at Cheyenne, Wyoming, in 1985.

An unusual summer weather system brought a severe storm, with heavy rains and hail, to our small, 126-bed general medical and surgical facility there on the evening of August 1st.

Only an hour after it started raining, a tremendous barrage of hail clogged storm drains surrounding the hospital. The continuous torrential downpour quickly built a standing water level in any depression around the building to a dangerous degree.

In a critical outside stairwell to the hospital's basement, the water level exceeded 7 feet, at which time the steel door crumpled, flooding the main bed building.

The hospital's elevator pits, several key basement equipment rooms and the auditorium were flooded to a depth of over 4 feet.

Simultaneously, the boiler plant doors gave way, and this key area was flooded to a depth of nearly 3 feet.

Many mechanical systems -- including telephones, main elevators, and all centralized computer applications -- immediately went out of service. Within an hour, the main power plant also had to be secured.

Emergency power quickly came on line, and very limited communications inside the facility were available through the security staff's radios.

The system for medical gases remained intact, and primary patient care was not affected. There was no immediate danger to patients or staff.

However, without hot water, air conditioning or complete lighting, the center took steps to reduce its census by temporarily discharging all non-acute patients, and by referring new admissions to other area medical facilities.

Full power was restored to the Cheyenne VA Medical Center two days after the flood, and the facility slowly began to build back to full operations.

Lessons learned from the experienced included:

- o That outlets and wiring for use of emergency power has to be thoroughly dispersed and well tested. It was discovered during the flood that the emergency generator did not activate lights in the center's nursing home, where nursing staff had to give medications by flashlight during the two nights under emergency power.

- o Backup files for the center's ADP operations should not all be kept in one place. These files, along with all computer hardware, were located in the basement, where they were a total loss.

4. Biloxi Hurricanes

Effects of flooding are only part of the consequences of another disaster VA has had extensive experience with: hurricanes.

Many of our facilities have sustained hurricane damage over the years, especially those near the Gulf of Mexico. But our Biloxi Medical Center holds the record for hurricane experience.

This southern Mississippi facility is dead center along the favorite track of hurricanes moving northwest from the Caribbean breeding ground.

Among those which have come ashore at Biloxi with notable result are Betsy, September 1965; Camille, August 1969; Frederick, September 1979; and Elena, September 1985.

All caused damage, but hurricane Camille is particularly well remembered. This storm slammed into the Medical Center with tremendous power, forcing a major evacuation, involving multiple airlifts to nine VA hospitals throughout the southeastern United States.

In 1969, this Medical Center operated nearly a thousand beds split between two divisions -- 209 general medical and surgery patients at the Biloxi Division, and 723 neuropsychiatric patients at the Gulfport Division. The latter division is located directly on the Gulf, separated by eight miles from the acute care building, which is inland.

First effects of hurricane Camille were felt on Sunday morning, August 17, 1969. Weather service warnings were not as sophisticated at the time, but there was little doubt this hurricane was to be a bad one.

By noon, main power at Gulfport was out and telephone lines were jammed. Strangely enough, the hospital couldn't contact local civil defense authorities, but could maintain telephone contact with VA Regional Headquarters.

The eye of the storm passed in late afternoon. At 7:00 p.m., the Gulfport Division Reported that the lights on the pier in front of the hospital had gone out. At 7:30, they reported the pier had gone, period. Within minutes, it was clear that motels and restaurants on the beach adjoining the Gulfport Division were being demolished.

In the Gulfport facility, surf battered into the first floor of many structures, including one patient building where patients and staff waited out the storm on upper floors.

As the storm receded the next day, two things were clear: first, miraculously, there were no casualties among the VA patient and staff population; and second, the Gulfport facility would have to be evacuated because of damaged buildings and complete lack of power, water and other sanitary necessities.

A huge evacuation program was mobilized, and -- over the next three days, 743 psychiatric patients were dispatched to nine VA Medical Centers throughout the southeast.

The task was undertaken by VA and what was then known as the military airlift command. Ground transportation and aircraft were furnished by the nearby Keesler Air Force Base.

VA Engineering and Administrative personnel worked to secure and clean up the Biloxi VA Center...

...While VA clinicians, nursing staff and volunteers worked with Air Force teams of nurses and medics to evacuate patients.

It's a real credit to this effort that not one injury to patients or emergency evacuation teams occurred.

The cleanup effort was huge and energetic. Within 30 days, all equipment was back in working order. Patients began returning to the Gulfport Division shortly thereafter.

Lessons learned were primarily in the context of emergency communications, and in making arrangements with other emergency forces for smooth evacuation procedures.

Emergency planning has advanced so far in the intervening years that it may not be beneficial to review specific actions taken during this episode. But the event does stand as a remarkable testimony to the power of hurricanes.

5. Grand Island Tornado

VA also has had experience with a natural disaster with similar damage potential, but offering less warning than hurricanes -- the tornado.

One of the most notable such events in our system occurred at our Grand Island, Nebraska, VA Medical Center.

6. Bay Pines Gas Leak/Denver Flood

The VA has had experience with another category of disasters as capable of destruction as the others we've been discussing. Since it doesn't seem quite fair to blame these on nature, we've called them "Human Inspired."

An example is the evacuation of our Bay Pines, Florida, Medical Center in 1982, after a backhoe digging a trench broke a natural gas main.

A more recent and better known incident, occurred at our Denver VA Medical Center, when millions of gallons of water flooded the sub-basement.

I do want to mention some interesting aspects to the Denver disaster which are different from several others we've experienced.

Initially, the Denver flooding did not seem particularly threatening.

Then the loss of water for drinking, general patient care, sanitation or food preparation became a concern. Some other medical support systems, such as suction, also ceased to operate.

Further dangers existed in having no water for fire sprinkler systems, and the possibility of losing electrical power. Since the main boiler system could only be run intermittently, the supply of heat also was limited.

Evacuation was undertaken, and it was conducted in excellent order, despite extremely cold weather conditions.

The Medical Center's Lobby became the natural place for "staging," during evacuation, with clinical staff assembling patients in this area before moving them out to ambulances in sub freezing temperatures.

With emergency teams, groups of administrative staff, ambulatory patients and news media also converging on this limited area, the lobby became extremely crowded.

This reflected the need for a command center during the emergency, which would have facilitated unrestricted access for staff and others with critical communications requirements.

During the period the Medical Center was closed for repairs, a command center was, in fact, established. This center proved vital in coordinating the care being given outplaced patients, and in communicating details about when the hospital would re-open, where staff should report, and where new patients applying for care should go.

The 229 evacuated patients were distributed among several area hospitals, most to the Fitzsimons Army Medical Center. The patients were returned five days later, after repairs had been made.

No injuries or deaths were sustained in the evacuation, but a significant proportion of the patient population experienced some adverse effects from the incident.

In the context of lessons learned from this incident, I would like to particularly take note of two observations:

First, communications were a problem. In this case, emergency communications radios were available, but, most hospital staff were inexperienced with radio operation and were slow and inefficient in using them.

Second, who would imagine that a nine story Medical Center -- located in the mile high city -- would have to contend with a flood.

Fortunately, sections of the facility's disaster plan describing evacuation procedures for fire emergency could be adapted to this situation.

The value of testing emergency equipment, and in maintaining flexibility in planning, is apparent.

7. San Fernando Earthquake

Returning to the event I began with, it's accurate to say that no disaster in the experience of the Veterans Administration has exhibited the power of the San Fernando earthquake, to influence policy and practice in emergency preparedness.

Within days of the incident, our VA Administrator toured the area with then Vice-President Spiro Agnew, Governor Ronald Reagan and Los Angeles Mayor Sam Yorty.

Not long afterwards, Congressional hearings were held to determine how to proceed in preparing for future earthquakes.

Studies coming out of these inquiries resulted in a major construction program for seismic reinforcements of VA Medical facilities in high risk areas.

The $500 million VA has expended on this effort since 1971 comprises the largest such seismic effort in the world.

Again, there's been so much progress in natural disaster planning since 1971 that it's of limited value to explore specific actions taken in the San Fernando disaster.

The two central buildings which collapsed housed some 90 patients taken by ambulance and helicopter to other VA hospitals in the area.

By noon of the day of the disaster, some 400 people -- including staff and volunteers -- were searching the ruins of the buildings. Two remarkable rescues took place many hours later.

One was a patient who had recently been removed from respiration therapy in an iron lung, but the apparatus had not been moved away from his bed yet.

The patient took refuge under the lung, and was rescued after several hours.

But the record for lengthy rescue went to an employee-- a 68-year old man who hid under a sink, and was rescued after 58 hours in the demolished building.

The San Fernando VA Medical Center no longer exists. The facility was determined to be too unsound to repair, and it was replaced by a new VA facility nearby.

But the experiences learned at the San Fernando facility live on in the disaster plans of all VA facilities in high seismic risk areas.

Observations

Some observations following a review of the VA's experiences with natural disasters are rather obvious, but worth stating.

In fact, two of these observations actually confirm current requirements of health care facility accrediting agencies. They are:

One, detailed plans must be developed to provide for effective response to natural disasters.

Two, these plans must be tested regularly.

These points mirror requirements of the Joint Commission on Accreditation of Hospitals.

The third point, which is not a requirement but equally valid, is that the response plans must be flexible.

All the elements in the rationale for these observations--implicit in the review of the selected natural disasters--need not be recounted here. But a few salient points can be quickly mentioned:

- Having a detailed plan provides a starting point for a systematic response.

  Even though it might seem to specify steps that would naturally occur to people in a disaster, there's value to such an instrument.

  It allows planners to think ahead to various contingencies, and affords managers the opportunity to consider--well in advance of a disaster situation--any special resources that should be procured and kept in readiness.

  Perhaps most importantly, it provides a quick reference for staff--in what may be confusing times--on what their responsibilities are and where their duty stations are.

- Testing such plans has obvious utility. VA Medical facilities around the country refine their disaster response time and technique through participation in regular tests with other facilities in the community.

One anecdote comes to mind, involving an emergency radio network established a few years ago to allow our California medical centers to communicate with each other and with regional headquarters in the event of a major disaster that might halt telephone service.

In this test, regional headquarters called three VA Centers on the dedicated emergency radio frequency, using equipment that is supposed to be monitored at all times. None of the three responded immediately on the radio.

One responded by telephone, saying they'd heard the call but did not know how to broadcast on the equipment.

After a telephone call to the second facility, where the equipment had been inadvertently switched off, they responded by radio. A third facility never responded at all.

The official conducting the test reported he wasn't able to reach that hospital at all during the test period, since--by coincidence--they also were having some switchboard problems.

Fortunately, this system has been upgraded since then, as has our ability to use it. But the point about testing is pretty clear.

Finally, the matter of flexibility. By definition, disasters are unpredictable. As we have seen, operations during full disaster mobilization can eventuate developments that don't turn up in tests.

For example, during the tornado in Grand Island, Nebraska, when we stopped air conditioning a utility area to conserve emergency power, we found that unfiltered dust particles caused shorts in the microprocessor circuitry in our lab equipment.

And in the incident involving our Denver VA Medical Center, flooding had never been imagined; and flexibility in the plan and in the thinking of those responsible for the evacuation made a good result possible.

The only answer to such unforeseeable events is to recognize, from the outset, that there must be flexibility in executing disaster plans.

CONCLUSION

The Veterans Administration has had extensive experience with natural disasters. Having reviewed representative instances, and having looked at current contingency planning, we believe our system is better able to respond to future natural disasters because of experience.

CHEMICAL HAZARDS ON SHIPS, ESPECIALLY TANKERS:

Toxicargo In General And Chemical Tankers

Chemical Hazards On Board

W.H.G. Goethe, Prof. Dr. med (ret)

Bernard-Nocht-Institute
Hamburg, Germany

Today, on practically all types of vessels there are risks through chemicals:

- o tankers,
- o gas tankers,
- o chemical tankers,
- o bulk carriers,
- o dry-cargo vessels,
- o container ships.

A great potential of danger exists on chemical tankers. By 1986, 861 chemical tankers were operating worldwide, carrying 3,560 million gross register tons, according to Lloyd's List. A great variety of products are being transported, sometimes one immediately after the other. They can be divided into the following groups:

- o petro-chemical products (e.g., mostly distillation and cracking products of refineries as paraffins, saturated and unsaturated hydrocarbons, different types of fuels, olefins, and lubricating oils).

- o coal tar products (e.g., aromatic compounds, benzene, toluene, xylene, phenol creasote and derivatives of these substances).

- o carbohydrate derivatives (e.g., different types of alcohols, methanol, propanol, aldehydes, etc.).

- o animal and vegetable oils (e.g. esters of different oils as glycerol, etc.).

- o heavy chemicals (a wide variety of most toxic substances can be transported; e.g., sulfuric acids, caustic soda, liquid sulfur, nitric acid, phosphoric acid, etc.).

Many of these substances can involve considerable toxicological dangers. The kind of intoxication can be acute or chronic, depending on the Cargo.

Health and Medical Aspects of Disaster Preparedness
Edited by J.C. Duffy
Plenum Press, New York, 1990

Main dangers arise during loading or unloading, when leakages or overflow, etc., occur. During the voyage, chemical accidents are very rare.

Mass cargo as well can cause dangers, especially during loading or unloading by producing dusts.

A lower range of dangers obviously exists on dry cargo and especially on container ships. Only some intoxications have been reported during loading or unloading, but here, accidents may happen caused by breakage of the cargo during the voyage due to bad weather conditions, wrong storage, or disasters at sea. Toxicological incidents on roll-on/roll-off vessels hardly ever occur during loading or unloading, but almost exclusively occur during the voyage by leaking tanks or by disasters at sea.

Numerous research programs on toxicological dangers to crews have been carried out in various countries. Most developed seafaring countries have dealt with this problem.

The main interest is clearly given to chemical tankers, followed by general purpose tankers. Results of very detailed research in this field can be found in Norway and Sweden.

OVERVIEW

1. The number of chemical accidents (intoxications and erosions) amount to only 1, 1% of all accidents recorded in German seafaring.

2. Regarding the causes of chemical, the following sequence is stated:

   a. intoxications by smoke or CO by fire on board
   b. intoxications by dangerous working materials, fuels or their derivatives.
   c. intoxications by dangerous cargoes.

3. Regarding the frequency of accidents related to the types of vessels, the following sequence is stated:

   a. chemical tankers
   b. tankers
   c. dry-cargo vessels
   d. mass cargo vessels
   e. container ships.

The high danger on chemical tankers is obvious, and on the other hand, the relatively high protection by container packing.

Which preventive and curative measures are necessary to avoid or lower the toxicological hazards/risks?

1. Regular, individual occupational medical examinations of seamen who regularly have contacts with chemical cargoes. This measure is taken in most seafaring countries. But only chronic damages can be traced here, never acute intoxications.

2. Best methods of ship construction and respective regulations, as they exist in national and international legislation, or as they are being prepared. Here, I should like to draw your attention to the intensive efforts by IMO in their Committee of Dangerous Cargo.

3. Shipmasters and officers have to be informed of the kind of danger deriving from each special cargo. This is an international problem not yet solved. When talking, e.g., to masters, ship officers and crew members of chemical tankers--running the highest risks--you will again and again find an amazing lack of knowledge regarding the toxicological dangers arising from their specific cargoes--inconceivable for a medical doctor. It is definitely a main task of shipping companies to keep masters with regard to the occupational health aspect.

4. According to IMO regulations, the forwarder has to take care that goods are properly declared according to:

   a. International Maritime Dangerous Goods Code (IMDG);

   b. Emergency Medical Services procedures (EMS); and

   c. Tables of Medical First Aid Guide for Use in Accidents Involving Dangerous Goods (MFAG).

   A special problem of the IMDG code is the "NOS (not otherwise specified) Position." For chemicals that have only a group identification but the compounds of which are unknown; e.g., "Pesticides NOS," obviously there can be no symptomatology and therapy stated. So far it has been impossible--in spite of all national and international efforts--to find out a useful procedure to solve this problem. We think it impossible, also, because it seems to be a question of squaring the circle. An immense number of chemical substances with totally contrasting toxicological features may be hidden in NOS items.

5. Special training of ship officers, and above all, of masters, regarding dangerous cargo; questions of occupational health care; working with measuring devices; test procedures, etc. Knowledge in this respect is very poor.

6. It is critical in case of a chemical accident that relevant information on the treatment of people be on board the vessel. Here we have to especially point to the Medical First Aid Guide (MFAG). The advantage of it is its easy handling and the fact that this guide is published in English and translations into other languages are available. The disadvantage is definitely the group tables that do not allow individual dealing with single toxic substances. This in any case is a "Prokrustes-bed." Individual tables per substance would be preferable, but they are difficult to prepare and do not exist in any country especially for shipboard use. The Federal Republic of Germany abolished its national information sheets after the MFAG had been introduced, as it was impossible to prepare tables for all existing substances.

7. In any case, toxicological additional equipment has to be on board any ship carrying dangerous cargo, as stated in MFAG, and in addition to the normal medical chest.

The main task for nautical medical doctors is definitely to take measures to prevent chemical accidents and intoxications on board. We should enlighten and inform masters, ship officers and crews in contact with or exposed to dangerous cargo to work together with all departments responsible for ship's safety.

In case of accidents that may happen in spite of all preventive measures, there has to be access to immediate information. It goes without saying that therapy is limited, but what is possible on board should be made available. We feel that radio medical advice will be necessary in most cases. At present, there is still a lack of knowledge as to which centers provide appropriate information and advice. Hopefully IMO will be able to produce a list of information centers worldwide which have a specific knowledge of the shipboard situation and the MFAG.

VETERINARY SERVICES IN DISASTERS AND EMERGENCIES

Arthur V. Tennyson, VMD

Director, Membership and Field Service
American Veterinary Medical Association
Schaumburg, Illinois

INTRODUCTION

Military personnel are quite familiar with disaster preparedness. Each military facility has a disaster preparedness plan that assigns tasks and responsibilities and allocates resources to deal with potential natural or man-made disasters that range from severe thunderstorms to nuclear warfare. We know that a clear plan is essential to immediate reaction, recovery from sustained damage, and moving ahead with our mission.

Few in the civilian community consider disaster preparedness. Wholesale destruction, mass casualties, complete utility failures, and interrupted food supplies are concepts seldom thought of. Police, fire, civil defense, and certain other government officials plan for us. They often have only limited input from other segments of the community. Without input from veterinarians, planners are liable to perceive only traditional, stereotypic roles for veterinarians. If so, veterinarians' capabilities and resources might be overlooked in the planning process and, for that reason, might not be used in a disaster. That would waste needed resources that could save and maintain lives that might otherwise be lost.

Veterinarians have a variety of skills and knowledge that might be essential to recovery in a disaster or emergency. Those resources must not be wasted. Veterinarians must make known their abilities and resources and participate in the planning process, so they will be included in the reaction team and accepted in the roles they can perform to aid recovery. Perhaps even more important, they must contribute from their expertise to assure complete and adequate planning in areas that might be overlooked without thoughtful contributions.

AVMA's Council on Veterinary Service addressed the problem recently in an attempt to update a 1963 document, "Veterinary Services in National Emergencies" (1), that was prepared in cooperation with the Departments of Defense; Health, Education, and Welfare; and Agriculture. The Council learned that most civil defense planning now occurs at the local and state level. To provide guidance for that planning, the Council sponsored a monograph, "Veterinary Services in Disasters and Emergencies," that was published in the Journal of the American Veterinary Medical Association (2). Reprints are available from the AVMA office, 930 North Meacham Road, Schaumburg, Illinois, 60196.

Health and Medical Aspects of Disaster Preparedness
Edited by J.C. Duffy
Plenum Press, New York, 1990

The monograph has three main purposes: 1. Establish in the veterinary literature, guidance for veterinarians who may need it in planning for and reacting to emergencies; 2. Motivate veterinarians to prepare for emergencies that could occur and to participate in civil defense planning in their communities; and 3. Awaken civil defense officials to veterinarians' capabilities as medical professionals and the need to include animal health care in their planning for disasters.

To accomplish those purposes, the Council selected veterinarians who are recognized authorities in their fields to prepare 12 papers that discuss major types of disasters for which we should be prepared. Each paper describes and discusses problems that are presented by the subject disaster and how veterinarians can contribute to resolving the problems. I will summarize some general concepts that prevail in disaster preparedness and how veterinarians can contribute.

The Threat

Throughout recorded history, mankind has been assailed with a variety of disasters of natural and man-made origin. History is punctuated with famines, floods, earthquakes, volcanic eruptions, and disease epidemics. Whole populations were wiped out in moments, as were the people of Pompeii when Mount Vesuvius erupted in 79AD and buried the city in ash. Such events seem only words in history books or subjects for costume movies of "ancient times," until, in 1980, the eruption of Mount St. Helens made it clear that such events can occur today and without warning unleash massive destructive power that almost defies the imagination. In 1986, a barrage of tornados marched through eastern Ohio, northern Pennsylvania, and southern Ontario leaving massive destruction in their wake. Those and similar events prove that disasters can occur any where, at any time.

We cannot prevent natural disasters. Seldom can we predict them with accuracy. We can only anticipate the probability and prepare in advance an organized, well thought-out response. In that way, all major participants can be aware of their responsibilities and prepare to carry them out with dispatch despite the chaos and confusion that prevails in the post disaster environment.

Natural disasters that have occurred in recent years have fortunately occurred in remote or rural areas with relatively sparse populations. They have been single events that affected a limited area and caused relatively few casualties. Disaster relief teams have been able to support survivors. Volunteer repair crews have cleaned up damage and helped rebuild. Medical relief teams from elsewhere have augmented local capabilities, and casualties have been transported outside the disaster area. There has been little threat to animal health in general, and veterinarians have not been greatly involved.

Some potential disasters could be so massive or so widespread that survivors will need to rely on their own resources for extended periods before outside help can reach them--if any outside help is available. Major earthquakes or nuclear or conventional warfare could be so widespread and create such massive destruction that they would make relief efforts difficult or impossible. Even well-planned terrorist attacks in multiple locations using chemical or biological agents could so disrupt the normal economy and medical care systems that they might prevent rapid response and relief to disaster areas. It is major disasters for which we must plan and in which veterinarians are most likely to be needed. If plans provide for the worst cases, we can apply those plans in a lesser degree for measured response to less serious situations. If a localized emergency arises, plans can be implemented to mobilize local resources immediately. If outside relief is available and more capable, so much the better. If not, we will be prepared to cope to the extent of available resources.

Planning for a major disaster must address a range of problems. They include:

1. Massive destruction of buildings, transportation networks, utility delivery systems, food and water supplies, and waste removal systems.

2. Large numbers of traumatic deaths and injuries of varying severity to people and animals.

3. Contamination of the environment and exposed personnel, foodstuffs, animal feeds, and pastures.

4. Confusion among survivors trying to find reason and hope amidst chaos.

5. Conflict among survivors competing for limited resources that threatens safety, order, and discipline.

6. Increased risk of disease in the absence of proper sanitation among depressed and debilitated survivors.

Such situations require organization and planning to coordinate relief efforts and maintain an orderly, disciplined response. Authorized relief forces must be identified in prior planning to assure they can obtain and use needed resources. Persons or groups that aren't part of recognized relief organization must be refused access to avoid misappropriation and black market distribution of scarce commodities. Government officials, police, fire, and military officials will be responsible to maintain order and discipline. Veterinarians and others must work within the framework of civil defense plans administered by those government agencies. We must assist civil defense officials to define veterinarians' roles in the plans. Then we must prepare to be able to carry them out.

Veterinarians' Roles

Most significant among activities in which veterinarians' education and training may be needed are: medical and surgical care of the injured, disease control and prevention, maintenance of animal health and preservation of food animals, inspection and approval or condemnation of food and water supplies, decontamination of recoverable foods and water sources, and proper storage and distribution of food and water. I'll discuss those activities briefly.

Care of Injured People

A major disaster will probably cause large numbers of dead and injured. The major earthquake expected to occur in southern California is anticipated to measure 9.5 on the Richter scale. An earthquake of that magnitude could cause tens of thousands of deaths and hundreds of thousands of injured within minutes. A nuclear war could cause untold numbers of casualties in an instant. Simultaneously, major medical centers may sustain major damage, reducing the existing medical care capacity. The demand for medical and surgical care could overwhelm the residual capacity of standard medical facilities to provide that care. Trained medical and surgical personnel will be urgently needed as will medical equipment and supplies.

Veterinarians have broad, general surgical training and experience oriented to several species of animals. In an emergency, they can and must care for one more species. The principles of medicine and surgery for humans and other animals are the same.

Most urban small animal practitioners perform surgery frequently, and most veterinarians have experience with severe traumatic injuries. Veterinarians who treat dogs injured in automobile accidents probably have more recent experience with traumatic injuries than most physicians who focus on medical rather than surgical practice. Veterinarians' surgical skills can save lives that might otherwise be lost for lack of available physicians to provide care.

Most veterinary hospitals are well equipped to provide surgical care. Veterinary hospitals are widely dispersed and are mostly one or two-story structures. They are more likely to survive in functional condition than are multi-story, central human hospitals. Fluids, instruments, anesthetics, antibiotics, and other medicines and supplies available in veterinary hospitals can be used to treat human patients.

Working with local physicians, or independently if necessary, veterinarians could assist in treating human casualties. Veterinarians can triage, control hemorrhage, treat shock, stabilize fractures, and clean, debride, and suture wounds. Where casualties are more numerous than physicians can handle, we can do more. In such situations, we must do all we can to help manage and care for patients and treat what we are able. We can, thereby, enable the available physicians and surgeons to concentrate on cases that most require their knowledge of human anatomy and diseases. Where human hospitals and other medical care facilities are able to accept patients, our goal should be to provide first aid and to stabilize the more seriously injured for transport to those hospitals. Where hospitals are destroyed or their capacity is overwhelmed, we must use our available resources to optimize care and make it available to as many people as we can.

In urban areas, care for injured animals will hold a lower priority than care for humans. We will have to deal with people who will insist that their pet dog or cat be treated. Our response will depend on the situation and the availability and need for services and supplies. Euthanasia of injured pets may be the only viable alternative.

The care of food producing livestock is another matter entirely and a serious one. Meat, milk, and eggs will be needed by survivors of the disaster. In the event of a nuclear, chemical, or biological war, there may not be outside food sources to replenish what is available in the local area. Food sources, especially livestock, must be conserved, and food products must be allocated according to need. If fuel supplies are disrupted, horses and other beasts of burden may become the only means of transportation and to accomplish work.

Rural veterinarians must keep the general welfare in mind as they respond to a disaster. With sparser human populations in their areas, rural veterinarians will not be as needed to treat human casualties, but they must address the injured and dead animals. The triage process must extend beyond the norm to deal also with animals that were killed traumatically. Veterinarians must decide among the injured which can suitably recover and remain productive and which cannot. That decision must consider the need for both immediate and long-range food supplies where refrigeration and other common preservation methods are limited or unavailable.

Animals that died traumatically must be evaluated to determine whether they can be safely eaten. If attended to within hours, such carcasses and other animals that must be slaughtered because of serious injury can be dressed and cooked to feed survivors of the disaster. Dead animals that cannot be consumed must be properly disposed to avoid their becoming a source of infection. Injured animals that can survive should be treated to prevent infection and bring about recovery. Such animals can best be preserved as a future meat source if they are kept alive for later slaughter. Animals that can recover to full production should be treated and preserved with those that are uninjured.

Public Health

Public health management is extremely important to the well-being of those who survive the initial disaster. In disaster environments, typhoid fever, cholera and other diseases abound. Vermin, whose normal habitats are disrupted by destructive forces, roam freely through the rubble spreading disease agents. Remains of dead people and animals provide a fertile source of pathogenic organisms. Water supplies are interrupted and often contaminated. The destruction of normal sewage and other waste disposal systems creates further risk of contamination of the environment.

Most of the United States populace knows little about survival in an adverse environment. The blessings we enjoy as one of the more advanced countries in the world could cause a serious disadvantage in a disaster environment. We have grown up with potable water running from our taps and fresh, safe, food available in every store. With few exceptions, we live in an environment that is clean and free of diseases that are common in crowded, dirty environments. Most haven't learned how to treat food and water to assure its safety and the need to keep the environment and food and water sources as clean as possible. As Lt. General Becton, Director of the Federal Emergency Management Agency, stated in an address on November 9, 1987, to the Association of Military Surgeons of the United States, "Our population is increasingly less self-sufficient."

It will be necessary to educate and guide survivors of a major disaster in essential sanitation and hygiene, as best they can be achieved in an austere environment without modern facilities and conveniences. Veterinarians can work with physicians, nurses, hygienists, and other knowledgeable people to establish an organized community sanitation program. They can then educate survivors on the requirements and their role in the public health program. People must be taught the consequences of poor hygiene practices, both as motivation, and so they can recognize and report early signs of breakdown or disease.

Once public health programs are organized, veterinarians can aid in monitoring and enforcing the programs and general sanitation measures. Their functioning as community public health officers will free other health professionals for other tasks. In addition, veterinarians, who are trained in herd health management (group health and preventive medicine), may be more attuned to the need than physicians who focus more often on the individual patient than the group. Veterinarians can design, implement and monitor preventive medicine practices, aid in immunization where vaccines are available, and recognize early signs of health deterioration. Where other medical care is unavailable, they can provide that care.

Animal Health and Preservation of Animals

The health of food-producing animals is especially important to longrange emergency planning. Human survival and welfare require that we preserve and protect agricultural livestock and assure a continuing supply of animal protein food products at a reasonable cost. Short-sighted evaluations and decisions in an acute situation could result in unnecessary loss and waste of food resources that, once lost, may not be replaceable for many generations, if at all. Preservation of breeding herds and flocks is essential to maintain a genetic pool of food producing species that can be used to re-establish a food production capacity.

Meat, milk, eggs, and their by-products are the major sources of dietary protein that is essential to growth, healing, and good nutrition. Animal-origin foods rapidly deteriorate if they are not properly preserved, stored, and prepared. Spoiled or contaminated foods can cause illnesses that may aggravate the disaster and impede recovery. Disaster planning must provide for controlled slaughter, rationing, security, and inspection to assure the availability, quality, and wholesomeness of foods for long-term as well as immediate survival. Implementation of those plans requires information and expertise to manage foods without electricity and refrigeration that may not be available in the post-disaster environment.

In a disaster, health care for pet animals depends on the situation and available resources. However, the human-animal bond is a strong one. Many pet owners consider their animals as family members that are entitled the same care, consideration, and chance of survival as any other family member. Whether disaster defense officials agree or disagree or can accommodate owner's concerns for pet animals, they must consider the importance of those concerns to pet owners. Such concerns may fuel resistance to actions that don't provide for evacuation or care of pets. Some people may refuse to evacuate without their pets. Those who survive without their pets may suffer grief and other psychological trauma, including guilt feelings for having abandoned their pets. Such reactions may interfere with their participation in or cooperation with protective or recovery activities.

Veterinarians, because of their education and training in animal anatomy, physiology, medicine, surgery, and epidemiology are most knowledgeable about the health and welfare of animals, and they are best able to make decisions regarding conditions that affect animal health. In a disaster or emergency, veterinarians can evaluate the effects on the health and welfare of livestock and pet animals and on the safety and quality of animal-origin foods.

Therefore, planning and implementing staffs of disaster teams should include veterinary officials in every government jurisdiction. Those veterinary officials should have direct access to decision-making authorities to present recommendations for animal health care and food management that are appropriate to the situation. Such input should be coordinated with the recommendations of human health care staff officials so the decision-makers may consider all aspects of the situation.

Inspection and Approval or Condemnation of Foods

In the immediate post-disaster environment, food may be plentiful, but subject to waste in the absence of electrical power, refrigeration, and other normal preservation methods. In the chaos and fear that prevails, people will tend to hoard food and, lacking knowledge of proper preservation methods, will probably waste a great deal. Foodstuffs in stores and warehouses will be vulnerable to damage and deterioration in the destruction of the buildings in which they are stored.

Depending on the severity and scope of the disaster, it may be necessary for governing agencies to commandeer and ration the issue of foods to the surviving populace. Such foods must be gathered quickly to avoid spoilage or looting. Foodstuffs must be inspected to condemn that which is hazardous, accept that which is safe and wholesome, and decontaminate that which is contaminated but recoverable. Veterinarians are probably best qualified to inspect and evaluate the safety of foods of animal origin. In the absence of other qualified inspectors in the average community, veterinarians are probably best able to evaluate other foodstuffs. Many veterinarians have served in the military veterinary corps and have specific training in food inspection.

Food Storage and Distribution

Proper storage must be provided for food to the extent that facilities are available. Canned goods should be sorted by type and stored in clean, dry secure areas if such are available so each type can be reached as it is needed. Vegetables and grains must be properly stored to maximize their shelf life. Perishables must be issued for early use to take advantage of their nutritional value before they spoil. Field expedient preservation measures should be employed to preserve meat and vegetables by canning, salting, drying, and smoking.

Veterinarians may serve in a supervisory capacity to assure proper treatment and storage of foods. They may also aid in calculating nutritional needs and advise on the rationed issue of available food to sustain the surviving population for the maximum possible time. Such issues can probably best be achieved with supervised central preparation and dining facilities that prepare measured portions for each person. Food hygiene and sanitation must be closely monitored in such facilities. Repeated inspection of stored foodstuffs will be necessary to detect and correct problems and prevent wastage.

Water supplies must also be monitored closely. Veterinarians who have small laboratories in their hospitals can perform bacteriological cultures of water samples in the absence of more sophisticated laboratories. Veterinarians as public health officials, or assisting them, can educate and advise people of the need and proper methods to boil or chemically treat contaminated water to make it safe to drink.

Veterinarians must also keep in mind and advise government agencies, producers, and the populace on the need to preserve and protect future food sources. Where involvement in the disaster is widespread, as in a nuclear war, each surviving community must ration stringently to preserve from each grain and vegetable stock enough of the best seed to plant next year's crops and assure the future food supply. Similarly, we must evaluate and select from among surviving livestock the hardiest and best producing individuals. Those animals must be preserved from slaughter. We must slaughter only those that we absolutely need to nourish the populace, and we must use every product of every animal to its maximum advantage. We must, if necessary, reduce ourselves to bare subsistence rations in the near term to assure that we and future generations will be able to eat next year and the years after. Veterinarians must evaluate the health and reproductive capacity of selected breeding animals and consult on their proper care and nutrition.

Many other concerns that might arise in disasters that veterinarians can address and where our training and expertise might be helpful to survival. We are a diverse profession with a wide variety of skills and expertise. Those abilities must be made known to the public and especially to the civil defense agencies who can plan for and use those skills in time of need. We must work together with civil defense planners at the local, state, and national levels to assure that in a disaster, veterinarians' skills and resources will be used where they are needed to contribute to the general welfare.

References

1. US Depart. of Agriculture: Veterinary Services in National Emergencies, Agricultural Handbook No. 255. U.S. Government Printing Office, 1963.

2. Veterinary Services in Disasters and Emergencies, edited by Robert J. Schroeder, DVM. Journal of the American Veterinary Medical Association, 1987; 190:701-799.

DISASTER PLANNING THAT ADDRESSES THE PRESERVATION OF CULTURAL PROPERTY

The Getty Conservation Institute
Marina del Rey, California

INTRODUCTION

On October 28 and 29, 1985, fifteen specialists in disaster planning for cultural property met in Los Angeles at the invitation of the Getty Conservation Institute. During the two days of meetings, the group evaluated the current state of disaster planning for both movable and immovable cultural property; identified the major problems in disaster planning, prevention, and response; considered means to heighten awareness of the need for disaster planning by the cultural heritage community and to communicate the conservation community's concerns to civil disaster planning authorities; and discussed ways in which the Getty Conservation Institute could support disaster planning efforts.

The meeting focused on natural disasters, such as floods, earthquakes, fires, tornadoes and hurricanes, and only briefly touched on man-made disasters such as terrorism. Security and problems caused by sophisticated technologies were also considered.

The group discussed conservation ethics and concluded that these often are in conflict with current preservation and restoration techniques. Proposed practices must be determined to be ethically sound before they are publicized and applied to cultural property.

Previous disaster planning initiatives were reviewed and the different needs of museum collections and historic structures were considered, as well as the political implications of a concerted, international attempt at determining standards for disaster planning worldwide.

Three major points were considered central to the issue of disaster planning for the cultural heritage:

1. Planning and prevention should be the first priority, with conservation treatment as the last resort;

2. A valuable collection belongs in a building designed to protect it;

3. Historic buildings follow the law of natural selection. A building that has survived for three hundred years may be better able than a more recent structure to withstand earthquakes. A list of specific recommendations follows.

Health and Medical Aspects of Disaster Preparedness
Edited by J.C. Duffy
Plenum Press, New York, 1990

RECOMMENDATIONS

During the course of the meeting, a number of recommendations were brought forward and discussed. These recommendations reflect activities that are needed by the field and are grouped in the following categories for presentation here: heightened awareness; resource development; information collection and dissemination; and scientific research.

I. Heightened Awareness

A. Communication with authorities outside the cultural property field

1. Collect and survey disaster planning literature published by civil and technical authorities. Identify areas in which basic information is needed to sensitize civil and technical experts to the needs of cultural property.

2. Attend conferences of disaster planning officials and present workshops on the special needs of cultural property.

3. Meet with representatives of the NSF, NAS, EERI, and other bodies to begin determining cooperative measures and common concerns.

4. Work with authorities to encourage the development of guidelines and building norms that best safeguard historic structures, collections, and modern museum buildings.

5. Organize a speakers' bureau to address targeted audiences; e.g., architects, engineers, scientists, fire departments, etc.

6. Develop a series of publications for these audiences that address the specific needs of different types of cultural property in various disasters.

7. Identify ways of communicating to key decision-makers the important ethical concerns regarding cultural property conservation.

B. Communication within the cultural property field

1. Planning must be the cultural property community's first line of defense, as conservation treatment should be viewed as the last step. Develop a short, concise document on disaster planning for administrators and other who set policy.

2. Develop contact with trustees and others with fiduciary responsibility for buildings and collections by working through risk management programs such as the NEA Indemnification Program.

3. Encourage senior management within museums to work with their local civil and technical authorities in developing disaster plans.

4. Develop general guidelines for establishing disaster plans so that museums can begin to institutionalize the preparedness and training of personnel.

5. Encourage ICOM to include disaster planning issues in the code of ethics.

6. Encourage signatories of the 1954 Hague Convention to consider adopting and implementing similar strategies for natural disasters.

II. Resource Development

A. Response tools

1. Determine how volunteer efforts can be integrated into existing response activities that are sponsored by groups such as UNESCO, EERI, NAS and FEMA.

2. Organize a roster of specialists who will be available to respond to disasters around the world.'

B. Planning tools

1. Develop a general handbook on how to plan for a disaster.

2. Develop materials that respond to specific needs within given regional jurisdictions.

3. Respond to needs of small museums by developing a manual on planning, response, legal rights, and appropriate restoration and conservation measures.

4. Commission the development of an annotated, computerized bibliography on disaster planning that includes civil, technical and cultural resources.

5. In cooperation with professional organizations, develop a survey questionnaire to identify planning activities in the field.

6. Organize a roster of specialists to consult with organizations concerning disaster planning. Encourage funding organizations that currently support conservation surveys of collections to also support disaster planning consultants.

III. Information Collection and Dissemination

A. Central repository of disaster planning information

1. Organize disaster plans in cooperation with existing international cultural bodies such as ICOM.

2. Survey and evaluate disaster plans that have been developed to date.

3. Establish a computerized file of disaster planning reports.

4. Collect documented damage assessments that are available through various organizations (engineers, architects, etc.).

5. Establish a central natural disaster planning office through an international body such as ICCROM.

B. Dissemination of Information

1. Identify ways to communicate new techniques and guidelines.

2. Develop a disaster planning bibliography for entry in the AATA database and create a disaster planning category in the hardcopy publication.

3. Computerize all information held in the central repository for dissemination through an organization such as CHIN.

4. Organize coverage of disaster planning activities in the newsletters of appropriate organizations.

IV. Scientific Research

A. Examine the recommendations from the 1985 ICCROM Skopje conference to determine areas requiring further research.

B. Investigate methods for measuring the effects of natural disasters so that planning and response measures can be developed and standardized.

C. Identify research areas related to disaster planning that need to be further developed.

D. Publicize the results of research related to disaster planning and response.

E. Develop standards on safeguarding historic structures and modern museum buildings in conjunction with civil authorities and engineers.

INTRODUCTION

The relationship of disaster planning to the cultural heritage is of general concern to the conservation community, both in the United States and abroad. "Museums for a New Century," a study commissioned by the American Association of Museums, identifies preservation of collections as a major priority. This area has suffered until now from a lack of follow-up to work done, communication problems both within the conservation community and between the conservation community and others concerned in disaster planning, and a lack of specific, easily-implemented recommendations for various situations. We must identify needs and specific actions that can be taken by the Getty Conservation Institute (GCI), either alone or with other organizations, to fill these needs.

Certain problems are central to the entire disaster planning issue. The first is that disaster response is too late; prevention must be the first priority. We must motivate reaction now and prevent overreaction after the event. This includes training and built-in structural and mechanical safeguards.

Relevant research for both prevention and response must be encouraged, publicized, and the results widely distributed; lay communities such as engineers and civil disaster planning/relief agencies must be involved and made aware of conservation issues; experts in disaster planning for the cultural heritage must be identified and their expertise made available worldwide; and effective communication must be maintained.

There is a need for planning and responding to natural disasters and only peripherally considered human or technological events such as arson, acts of terrorism, vandalism, or crises brought about by the failure of sophisticated equipment or by the contamination of water tables by sewage. The primary preventive measure in most of these latter events is security, not disaster planning per se, and the results (fire in the case of bombing, for example) require the same response as disasters with natural causes.

It has been noted that "all disasters end in flood" (whether by tidal wave, hurricane , broken pipes, or fire-fighting) and that the majority of fires in cultural institutions are the result of construction or other work that affects electrical systems. Arson is rarely intended specifically to destroy artifacts and is instead often politically motivated, as in the fire-bombing of John F. Kennedy's birthplace, or because the cultural institution is seen as symbol of wealth or authority in a poor or disaffected society.

There are a number of roles the GCI might play. These include sponsoring periodic meetings on disaster planning to maintain awareness and facilitate communication; developing a roster of specialists available in case of disaster; using its newsletter to disseminate information on disaster planning resources and techniques; and providing for the collection, publication, or computerization of information resources. Research via the Institute's Scientific Research Program is also a possibility.

ETHICS

Preservation Techniques

The ethics and philosophy of disaster planning for the cultural heritage do not change; only the technology does. These ethics often conflict with current techniques for the preservation of cultural property. It it important to preserve the interiors of historic buildings, not just the facades; often so much work is done on an interior that only the facade remains. The use of reinforced concrete may not only destroy the integrity of the building but may also further weaken the structure. Some of the historic buildings in Mexico that suffered the worst damage during the recent quake were those that had undergone some sort of restoration or reinforcement. Other techniques, such as the heating and humidifying of old buildings to provide appropriate environments for art objects and humans, may also damage the structure.

Ironically, the structures we cherish most are often the first to receive drastic treatment, precisely because of our concern with preserving them. As a result, they often suffer the worst consequences when the next disaster strikes. The technical knowledge is available but the principles of applying this knowledge rarely find their way to the decision-makers. Conservation technology needs to be carefully examined and evaluated before it is publicized or applied.

Overreaction to Disasters

Many factors contribute to the tendency to overreact to disasters. In many countries, the architect's fee is a percentage of the cost of the building work to be undertaken, encouraging the use of greater rather than lesser measures. Often great amounts of aid money are available after a disaster, which may also encourage inappropriate techniques. In many cases the people responsible for deciding whether buildings should be demolished after a disaster are not trained in cultural heritage preservation and have little idea of the cultural value of historic structures. It is vital to get across to administrators and civil authorities both the technical _and_ the cultural aspects of such decisions.

Conservation Ethics in Disaster Planning

Conservation ethics dictate the least possible intervention. Studies are being done on the life expectancies of various materials. While wooden structures and historical structures in quake areas are obviously at critical risk, we have little choice about materials in many cases--we must work with what we have. We do have control over materials used in display and storage;

both the GCI and the Canadian Conservation Institute are working on studies of these materials.

Three major points emerged as central to the ethics of disaster planning: one, prevention and planning must be the first concern, as conservation is the last step; two, put the valuable collection in a building that can protect it; and three, the law of natural selection operates in quake areas.

THE STATE OF THE ART: DISASTER PLANNING RESOURCES

The conservation community needs, first, to be aware of the resources already existing in the disaster planning field. Many of these resources are underused or not used at all, when they might contribute considerably to preserving the cultural heritage in case of natural or man-made disasters. Conference proceedings go unpublished because of a lack of funding; other information that is available is not widely distributed. Issues such as a definition of what constitutes cultural property, varying definitions of what constitutes cultural property, varying concepts of restoration, and means to communicate new techniques and guidelines must be resolved before efforts can be effective.

International Efforts

The major international cultural heritage organizations all have some involvement in disaster planning. ICCROM is preparing a handbook for those responsible for historic structures, and will be distributing Sir Bernard Feilden's handbook, "Between Two Earthquakes" (with particularly heavy distribution in the Mediterranean area) as part of a series. They publish abstracts, have in their library approximately 200 publications on earthquakes, and have collected information on the behavior of various structures. An ICCROM research project has resulted in an exhibition on earthquakes and a bibliography, now linked with the Smithsonian Institution. They see a need both for general handbooks and for studying specific needs in different regions.

ICCROM's policy is to assist any member state which requests aid in the event of a disaster. ICCROM member states should be asked to have national disaster planning offices or commissions to help disseminate information supplied by ICCROM.

ICCROM recently sponsored a conference in Skopje which resulted in recommended measures to be taken for the protection of cultural property. It was suggested that these recommendations could be the basis for research through the GCI's extramural research program. These recommendations will be presented to the ICCROM Council and the General Assembly.

The ICOM Security Committee tries to get information from quake countries after the event, generally with little success. The possibility of a Working Group within the ICOM Conservation Committee, which would be in a position to produce guidelines and (possibly) recommendations for governments, was suggested. The ICOM code of ethics, now in its second draft, currently does not include disaster planning. This issue will be brought up before the finalized code is presented at the General Conference.

ICOMS had an international committee on earthquakes for six years. It was abolished in 1985 and reformulated as the Structural Problems Committee. The last chairman proposed was Sir Bernard Feilden.

Two United Nations organizations, UNESCO and UNDRO (United Nations Disaster Relief Organization), are involved in disaster planning. UNDRO publishes literature on disaster planning, including bibliographies.

The 1954 Hague Convention on the Protection of Cultural Properties in the Event of Armed Conflicts outlines a system by which culturally important buildings could be identified in advance, then classified by the degree of damage suffered. It also provided guidelines for determining the historical and cultural significance of various buildings. Any signatory to the convention is supposed to have done such a cultural property inventory. Though the system was intended for use in wartime, it would work equally well in natural disasters. Yugoslavia's inventory, done according to this system, helped greatly in documenting the damage after the Montenegro earthquake. Accurate records and maps also save time and effort in deciding where to go and what to work on. This effort must be made nationally, not just for specific buildings.

Resources at the National Level

Individual countries also have private and governmental bodies working either directly or indirectly in the disaster planning field. Much of this structure could be used in creating any comprehensive disaster plan for cultural property, and also in disseminating information. For example, Switzerland and Germany sponsor Technical Aid Communities, teams of volunteers who do both assessment and rescue work in case of disaster. These teams often include conservators as well as disaster relief workers.

The Canadian Conservation Institute deals with the average of 5 major disasters a year. These are occasions when it is necessary to send someone from CCI to the disaster site. In addition, they advise people on smaller crises by telephone at least 20 times a year.

With support from the U.S. government's National Science Foundation (NSF), the National Academy of Science (NAS) through its Committee on National Disasters and the private Earthquake Engineering Research Institute (EERI) operate teams similar to the European Technical Aid Committees. The Committee on National Disasters is on call worldwide and publishes reports of its missions after each disaster. Similarly, the EERI sends out reconnaissance teams to earthquake areas. Unfortunately, both organizations deal only with damage to buildings and people, and not with damage to cultural property. It was suggested that the cultural heritage community become involved in these emergency response teams so that information about cultural property will be included in reports and publications and so that the conservation community can have access to data collected by these organizations.

The National Bureau of Standards of the U.S. government also does work relevant to disaster planning; for example, flammability studies. Computer models have been developed by Harvard University which can determine the disaster planning requirements of specific museums and can make both predictions and recommendations on cost-effective measures. Other U.S. government resources are the Federal Emergency Management Agency, the National Endowment for the Arts, and the National Parks Service. It is suggested that people involved in these and similar efforts be included in the conservation community's discussions.

The U.S. government has a national disaster plan. This term refers specifically to disasters affecting a large part of the country. Although it is intended primarily for the use of federal agencies in case of war, it does define cultural heritage, sets forth policy, and allocates responsibility. The President must declare a national disaster before the plan can be put into effect; it is under the supervision of the Federal Emergency Management Agency. It is suggested that contact with the FEMA could be very helpful and that the GCI function as a liaison with that agency.

Relevant work is also being done by organizations in other countries; for example, the British engineering community has compiled architectural guidelines for renovating historic structures. It was suggested that the Research Institute of the American Institute of Architects and the National Bureau of Standards might be willing to compile a comprehensive text. It is important to determine whether this would be general material, useful over wide geographical areas, or whether it would have only regional application. A short paper might be preferable to a book. The work needs to get to quake-prone areas in spite of the existing codes in individual countries.

The EERI has a committee similar to Japan's committee on the anticipated Tokyo earthquake, which may now be encouraging preparedness committees and looking at society's responses to all disasters, not just earthquakes. It was suggested that conservation-minded speakers address EERI meetings.

Other professional organizations not normally thought of as conservation-related often in fact conduct work directly applicable to cultural heritage preservation. The Structural Engineers Association of California sets standards for building codes in the state, which influence all the building codes in the U.S. The U.S. codes, in turn, have worldwide influence. Heightening the cultural awareness of engineers so that cultural property issues are considered in establishing building codes might have far-reaching effects.

Publications

Numerous publications exist, some dealing specifically with cultural heritage and others dealing with civic disaster planning which could be useful. Bernard Feilden's book, "Between Two Earthquakes," has already been mentioned; other publications include "Earthquake Effects and Protecting Museum Artifacts," the British guidelines and building codes mentioned above (although building codes may sometimes be the enemy of historic structure rather than the saviour), and the books "Museum Security" (ICOM) and "Museum, Archive, and Library Security." The University of Colorado publishes a newsletter, the "National Hazards Observer." "AATA," already online, is a potential tool for wider dissemination of this material and there was discussion of adding a disaster planning section to it. Other suggestions for publications included the commissioning of an annotated bibliography and development of a thesaurus on cultural heritage.

Professional Meetings

The results of other meetings on disaster planning are also of interest. In March 1982 a meeting on "The Protection of Historic Architecture and Museums Collections from Earthquakes and other Natural Disasters" was sponsored by the National Science Foundation in Washington, D.C.: the papers, directed at museum boards and decision makers, were published in the spring of 1986. A meeting on "Emergency Planning for Museums, Galleries and Archives," organized by the British Columbia Provincial Museum in October 1984, produced papers which have been be published.

COMMUNICATION: A VITAL TOOL

The conservation community urgently needs to communicate its priorities and requirements to the many people and organizations involved in disaster planning. In this context it is important to understand how the perspectives and priorities of civil disaster authorities and the cultural property interests differ.

Civil Authorities

Governments are often ill-equipped to efficiently save lives, let alone museum collections. In a major disaster, civil resources will be devoted to human needs; in a minor disaster affecting only the cultural property, civil authorities are not mobilized. The allocation of precious resources to inanimate objects when people are suffering is a serious public relations problem. Local resources, such as fire and police departments, protect lives first and property second. In addition, "property" to a firefighter means the building, not the building's contents. Many are very surprised to discover that the contents of a museum are more valuable than the structure itself.

Dependence on civil relief, therefore, is a major problem of priorities and ultimately the responsibility must rest with those in charge of cultural property. Because help may not be the conservation community's first line of defense. Thus it is essential to maintain close contact with local authorities and ensure that they are familiar with both the structure and the collection. This can be of great help in minimizing both fire and water damage. Firefighters in Turin, for example, have different plans for fighting fires in different parts of the cathedral. It is also useful for conservators to become fire wardens at their institutions; in this way they are among the first to be admitted after a disaster. The local authorities should in any event have a list of people, conservators or others, to be admitted after a disaster. Museums need supplies on hand and day-to-day precautions such as the tying down of objects in quake-prone areas.

Earthquakes also create a need for speedy access to buildings. Much damage occurs in the few days after a quake as buildings are bulldozed to prevent their collapse. The people who make these decisions are rarely trained in cultural heritage preservation; they are held responsible if lives are lost and thus when in doubt will usually opt for demolition. Conservators can sometimes be most effective by not going through channels, which can cause costly delays. "Get there fast and look official" is suggested as a way of getting access in many circumstances.

Cultural Organizations

Even people involved in the museum world are sometimes unaware of the need for disaster planning. Major disasters like earthquakes come so rarely that it is next to impossible to maintain a high level of readiness. Constant changes in personnel can make training a major financial burden. To offset these problems, museums need to institutionalize the preparedness and the training of personnel. The museum's physical plant and its administration must provide a system for making preparedness and mitigation measures self-perpetuating. Anything that leads to easy access is, in effect, disaster planning. The act of creating a disaster plan can be very important in itself, and planning for a major disaster will enable an institution to cope with routine situations which often cause more damage in the long run.

With limited resources, museums must put their money where it will have the most effect and remember that a disaster is an emergency that got out of hand. In prevention, this means that architects, designers, boards, and directors must be convinced to build in precautions whenever possible. A well-prepared presentation to architects, planners, and museum directors was suggested as a way to achieve this; it might be a collaborative venture between the GCI and ICCROM.

The more complex the institution, the more chance there is that something will go wrong with systems such as fire prevention. Sophisticated systems are also vulnerable to power failures, which can be caused by conditions hundreds of miles away. For example, the National Museum of African Art in Washington, D.C., will be located in a basement. Because of the high water table in the D.C. area, it will be under water if the pumping system fails. Canada's National Museum of Man, on the other hand, can evacuate and seal its building in a quarter hour to preserve the humidity if its air conditioning system stops functioning. Such a rapid response requires that one person have the authority to make the decision without going through channels.

Many small local museums and historical societies have given little or no thought to disaster planning. The same layout is used time and again in many different buildings. This audience needs information as much as the larger museums do; existing publications are not widely known Resources needed include a do-it-yourself manual on disaster planning to lead museum administrators through the planning process; information on responding to a disaster, determining a building's stability, and stabilizing it; information on the legal rights of owners and museums; and information and the appropriate measures to take in doing repairs. It was suggested that the curator of a small museum does not need an involved technical paper; a simple publication that spells out the problem, makes judgments, and draws conclusions may be preferable.

Accountability

Accountability is an issue in many cases. Who takes the responsibility to institute protective systems? Smoke detectors in the attic of the Roosevelt home in Hyde Park were estimated at $2,000; the decision not to install them resulted in $2 million worth of damage. It is also important to convince trustees of their fiduciary responsibility for the building and its collections. In New York state, museum directors and trustees are being legally liable for the safety of their collections. A catalogue of disasters since 1970 impress museum directors with the seriousness of the problem.

Insurance also touches the disaster planning issue. Insurance companies should be excellent sources of information about what has been claimed, and they often have considerable influence on precautionary measures; for example, New York State requires all museums to have sprinkler systems in the galleries. However, the insurer's definition of success and failure may differ considerably from the conservator's. For example, the insurance industry considers a sprinkler-head failure to be a time when the sprinkler does not go off. The conservator, on the other hand, considers it a failure when it goes off for no reason. The conservation community needs to make its voice heard in insurance legislation and the different measures people may take to satisfy both insurance and conservation needs (for instance, halon systems to extinguish a fire before it sets off the sprinklers).

The NEA indemnification program for foreign exhibits is a source of good information. It was suggested that a disaster plan be made a requirement of the indemnification for the loan of an exhibit and that the program be expanded to the national level.

Ultimately, museum administrators will set the priorities. Disaster planning can be made a showcase item, as conservation has come to be in recent years. Information on the needs of individual collections and the available resources can be used to convince a board of trustees or a large donor to act. Few museums now have even simple plans; publicity about what an earthquake or other disaster can do and an effective presentation to a board of trustees might encourage greater preparedness among both administrators and conservators. Japan has recently gotten excellent results from preparedness campaigns, and Finland has held a conference for the Directors General of government agencies on the conservation of historic buildings.

This kind of training raises the awareness of the civil authorities, and thus encourages buildings norms that favor sound conservation practice. Such seminars must be focused for specific audience. The Feilden handbook, which is primarily intended for administrators, could be supplemented by slides. A speakers' bureau of experts could talk on specific topics to museum directors, library associations, architects planners, historical preservation programs, legislatures, etc. The GCI might arrange this service and assist the speakers in preparing appropriate materials.

Little information is available on how to protect objects; usually the focus is the building. Once this information becomes available, people must be encouraged to act on it. Often people take measures that cut such costs as insurance premiums, and what saves lives often conflicts with what saves collections. The GCI should pinpoint specific museums, invite the decision-makers, and present them with a short, concise, to-the-point document.

Special Needs of Historic Structures

Historic buildings give rise to different issues than contemporary museums, and there are further difference between historic buildings housing a collection and historic buildings alone. Measures like climate control and humidification taken to protect a collection installed in a historic building may be good for the collection but bad for the structure. For these reasons, buildings in undeveloped areas may be better off from a preservation standpoint than buildings in highly developed areas. Norms must distinguish between contemporary museum buildings and historic buildings; this information must be disseminated and the fear of disaster kept alive. Regular inspections and contact with museum directors can accomplish this.

It is a mistake to focus on only one form of disaster (fire, earthquake). One man's quake-proof styrofoam packing is another man's fire hazard. There are chemical risks to a collection from fumes, gases, etc. regardless of the type of disaster. CCI is involved in materials testing in this regard.

Need for Additional Information

Many existing publications now go to the same small group of people who attend disaster planning meetings; they are not reaching the rest of the community. Different types of cultural property require different measures and guidelines and thus separate publications are needed. A series of publications would be necessary; one problem is determining priorities.

Finding out what has already been done is a major problem. Existing literature on disaster planning needs to be organized, critiqued, abstracted, and included in bibliographies, and this information needs to be accessible to the cultural heritage community. An annotated bibliography could be the beginning of an ongoing collection and updating of data. Civil disaster planning literature should also be included; though it is sometimes only incidentally concerned with cultural property, plans developed for dealing with nuclear power plants, toxic wastes, etc. contain much information. This, of course, requires an organization that has the staff and funding to support such an operation on an ongoing basis.

Regardless of specific subject, the publications should all include the following:

Illustrations of good examples (i.e., appropriate materials and actions), from conception to execution.

Policy and principles for the decision-makers.

A practical handbook of appropriate measures, dealing both with mitigation and with the after effects of a disaster. This may already exist and that information may be available in critical abstracts.

Need for Increased Awareness and Cooperation

Any new tools produced will be useless without a corresponding awareness. The conservation community itself must take a broader view than it normally does and remember that disaster preparedness is more than planning; it also includes specific mitigation measures to avert disaster. This will require an established, easily implemented program for museum collections. Another part of this process is documenting the need for disaster preparedness and the interaction of events which occur during a disaster. Efforts first must focus on a limited number of museums until the credibility of specific approach has been established. It can then be standardized on an internal level and will eventually "trickle down" to the smaller museums.

This of course requires government cooperation, in order to avoid the undermining of standards by legislation in individual countries. How can civil disaster planning measures be applied to cultural property? The GCI must communicate the ethics of cultural property conservation to the key decision-makers and act as liaison with other disaster planning groups. A short publication mailed internationally to the boards of trustees of all museums would be important.

Decisions about disaster planning must come from senior management; they are beyond the authority of conservators. Usable material needs to be developed and directed at museum directors, along with motivational material and directives for those actually carrying out the plan. A series of meeting over several years and a series of workshops for museums directors, conservators, and security staff can be important. The emphasis should be on useable materials, not research and meetings. Disaster planning should be discussed at large general meetings, rather than within small groups, to include the people who "should be there but aren't."

It is also important to communicate research results that affect disaster planning and response. Publicizing research programs would provide a basis for comparison and would also help to reach specific audiences; for example, some institutions are studying proper ways to reinforce buildings, but their findings are not being communicated to the engineering community.

A small traveling exhibition for curators and directors on how to prepare displays in seismic areas would be valuable. Great care must be taken in making specific suggestions, however, as different geographic areas react differently to quakes. The use of museum education departments to help people plan for the safety of objects in their homes is an important role.

RESPONSE TOOLS

Political Considerations

Any concerted effort to increase disaster preparedness in the cultural heritage community must consider the effect of national and international politics on the issue. At UNESCO's General Conference in 1983, many member states were opposed to the idea of adopting a Convention for the prevention of the effects of natural disasters. National sovereignty and the fear that foreign relief teams could be used to disguise other activities were among the reasons for such opposition. At most an international decision can only be a catalyst. Even when the network is non-political, there can be serious political and psychological obstacles to gaining access to many countries.

Any attempts to organize disaster planning worldwide must first be on a non-governmental basis since a neutral effort with no government ties can more effectively determine people's response capabilities. It was suggested that this effort be discussed with the international conservation organizations. Groups or individuals working in the field need contact with ICCROM, ICOM, ICOMOS, UNESCO, EERI, etc. to determine how volunteer efforts can be integrated into disaster relief plans.

It is also important to separate training from assistance. First build learning; then offer help.

Disaster planning requires an order of priorities which can only be determined on the national level. Each country must be responsible for its own inventory of cultural property (which is generally lacking) and any instructions or regulations concerning it. These national regulations then need to be placed in an international context, which may perhaps encourage individual countries to act.

But the national and institutional focus will be different from country to country. Each museum will have different plans and priorities for its collection.

Central Information Repositories

Response tools fall into two general categories. The first is information. Central respositories of disaster planning information, duplicate collections catalogues in safe places, and bibliographies are important. A central repository, for instance, would encourage museums to develop a disaster plan, provide access to other institutions' plans for purposes of comparison, and provide information to relief agencies when a disaster occurs. Such a central resource might be online with the Canadian Heritage Information Network. A questionnaire to determine what aspects of disaster planning institutions have considered would have the additional value of pointing out areas needing to be addressed further. This could first be used to create awareness of the issue and then be converted into specific recommendations for follow-up by various organizations such as the American Association of Museums and the American Association for State and Local History.

In terms of other information tools, a bibliography is the most easily created. Getty may support the preparation of a bibliography to be included in an online database. Create a new category of AATA . In addition, the GCI newsletter could publicize the needs for disaster planning and explain to the community any actions the Getty is taking.

A roster of specialists on disaster preparedness who can provide information and/or assistance to individual countries is another possibility. In the past, people involved in such efforts have been primarily structural engineers. A method for preparing such a roster would have to be devised. People with the appropriate expertise need to be located, contacted, and provided with information and other resources.

Response Teams

This or other group of specialists might also function as response teams in disasters. Such a team might include archaeologists, ethnographers, conservators, historians, or other appropriate specialists. An internationally accepted individual is better able to assess damage and give advice. The teams would build up case records, develop a cadre of experts familiar with the effects of disasters, evaluate appropriate prevention and response measures, and assess long-term needs for assistance. The teams might be structured in such a way that the first team, drawn from the roster of specialists, could assess a situation and call for an appropriate second team. A mechanism is also needed to coordinate volunteers and maintain contact with the many agencies involved in disaster relief.

These teams might meet annually, hold special meetings in response to specific disasters, or meet more frequently until they are well established. The meetings would be held in different parts of the world to enable the teams to maintain contact with colleagues in different countries and have access to information on specific disasters. The organizational body consist of a core staff and an **ex officio** board representing major organizations. Funding could be requested from the NEA, NEH, and similar organizations.

These teams also offer an evaluation of preventive measures in individual institutions which might be eligible for funding under the J. Paul Getty Trust Grant Program's provision for surveys of the conservation needs of permanent collections. The groups could also organize a certain number of activities at the regional, national and international level aimed at decision-makers, and function as a training and consulting body.

In view of political considerations, agreements could be made in advance with individual countries for this team's assistance in the event of disaster, since waiting to be asked can result in considerable delays.

If such a roster and group were formed, the GCI newsletter could advertise their existence and explain their capacity. The roster itself should also be made available so that countries could contact individuals directly.

Planning for Specific Disasters

Specific problems relating to different types of disasters also need attention. For example, overreaction to earthquakes can lead to renovations of existing structures which actually do more harm than good. Studies are being conducted in Milan, Florence, Salerno, and Yugoslavia; certain institutions are experimenting with the grouting of historic structures or collecting information on the behavior of various types of buildings which need different conservation measures. Research along these lines needs to be continued and publicized. Also, the geological condition of the area needs to be assessed; the Skopje conference put little emphasis on seismic testing.

The success of disaster planning in individual institutions depends on availability of staff to execute the plan in such situations. Since staff members must first be assured that their families are safe, telephone communications must be kept open. Air conditioning systems must continue functioning, which in turn may require an independent power source.

Much needs to be done if we are to guarantee the future of our cultural heritage from the ravages of natural and man-made disasters.

A REVIEW OF MEDICAL RESPONSE TO DISASTER CASUALTIES

Douglas A. Rund, M.D., FACEP

Associate Professor and Director
Ohio State University
Columbus, Ohio

SUMMARY

This chapter summarizes a review of medical response to disaster casualties. The goals are the following:

(1) to develop a hypothetical model for investigating the health and medical aspects of disaster preparedness;

(2) to determine investigational areas most critical to the health and medical aspects of international disaster care planning;

(3) to identify available medical data on specific injuries and illnesses associated with particular types of disasters;

(4) to begin collection and analysis of specific disaster plans for the United States and NATO countries.

By studying disaster reports of recent years, one may be able to compile types and magnitude of injuries and illnesses expected in specific types of disasters and measures taken in disaster care. In such a fashion we could develop strategies for anticipating health and medical needs in specific disasters, and assessing such needs in the affected areas based on early data from the disaster areas. In light of such findings I will be examining the emergency medical response portion of the disaster plans of NATO countries to determine areas that require further development, and to determine when and what kind of international aid may be necessary. I would also like to present an outline for projects requiring coordinated international effort such as developing a coding scheme for medical equipment and supplies, a standardized strategy for early mobilization of appropriate experts, and effective operating procedures for developing a system for proper international response.

INTRODUCTION AND DEFINITION

While it is difficult to offer a single, comprehensive definition of "disaster," some delineation of the boundaries of this term, in its common usage, may be of value. Disasters are unexpected events which have the potential of causing mass casualties and overwhelming the coping mechanisms

Health and Medical Aspects of Disaster Preparedness
Edited by J.C. Duffy
Plenum Press, New York, 1990

of the community. The disasters are caused by particular "agents" (earthquake, flood, radiation, toxic substance, tornados and storms, and a great variety of other natural events or the products of human actions and inventions). The key feature is the overwhelming nature of the event, swamping resources for dealing with potential casualties. Clearly, assessment of the physical and social consequences of such events in their specific settings and the application of methods for coping with such consequences are the key dimensions.

Recognizing the need for specific definitional criteria, particularly from a medical point of view, the International Trauma Foundation established a working party in 1980 that produced a report submitting the following definition: "A disaster is a destructive event which, relative to the resources available, causes many casualties, usually occurring within a short period of time."(1) This definition includes five specific components quite useful in helping to label specific events as disasters: 1.) the event itself; 2.) the destructive nature of the event; 3.) resources available to manage the effects of the destructive event; 4.) casualties disproportionate to the extent of available resources; and 5.) a time frame.

With regard to the event itself, a major distinction can be made between naturally occurring events and man-made events, thus creating two categories. Table I lists types of disasters classified in each category. Although such a list is not exhaustive, it is reflective of events commonly encountered throughout the world.

The destructive nature of the event, at least with regard to environmental emergencies, has been classified by Irey.(2) He divides such events into four classes: 1) physical (including mechanical, thermal, radiation, and electrical; 2) chemical (including human exposure by accidental spill, vaporization or contamination; 3) biological (epidemics associated with disease-producing organisms); and 4) psychological (including states or panic and hysteria generated by all of the physical, chemical or biological types of emergencies).

A third component of the proposed definition involves resources available to meet the needs generated by the disaster. Although Rutherford et al., have proposed the terms "simple" and "compound" to distinguish disasters that do not disrupt rescue and medical care capability of the systems (simple), from those that do disrupt such capabilities (compound); such distinctions rarely apply to disasters requiring international medical response where, almost by definition, the needs generated by the event exceed the resources locally available to manage the casualties. Types of resources needed for proper medical responses to disasters are included in Table II.

The fourth component of the definition includes the number of casualties resulting from the disaster. Some reports have justified the term "disaster" if the number of casualties exceeds the arbitrary number 25.(3) However, some systems are capable of easily handling 25 seriously injured persons. Consequently, the proposed definition that the number of casualties exceeds the capability of the system and calls for additional resources, seems more appropriate and certainly more generalized.

Many reports of disasters have shown that one of the primary problems in immediate disaster relief aid is the inability to rapidly quantify the extent of disaster, types of health and medical needs, and the ready availability of resources to the needs. From a review of published data that we have conducted thus far, we find it difficult to estimate the numbers of or types of casualties to be expected from a specific type of disaster, even allowing for different settings. Perhaps reflecting this obvious lack of precise data is the rather arbitrary classification of disasters proposed by the International Working Party (4) in 1980:

1.	Minor	25-100 10-50	casualties alive or dead, or casualties requiring hospital admission
2.	Moderate	100-1000 50-250	casualties alive or dead, or casualties requiring hospital admission
3.	Major	more than 1000 more than 250	casualties alive or dead, or casualties requiring hospital admission

The fifth component of the definition includes the time factor. Most events commonly considered to be disasters occur suddenly, unexpectedly, and at unpredictable times and places. Although the term "creeping disaster" has been used to identify certain slowly developing disasters such as famine or drought. Another rather arbitrary classification regarding time is: short (less than one hour), relatively long (between one and 24 hours), and long (greater than 24 hours).(5) It may be useful to develop such a scale on the basis of empirical data.

The available literature and our common experience make it possible for us to formulate a working definition of disaster that takes into account the health and medical needs and that may be subdivided into individual components convenient for additional study or analysis. As stated earlier, data about types of injury or illness associated with specific disasters are difficult to derive from the literature. As an example, we know that an earthquake in Guatemala caused the following categories of injury: laceration and crush injury caused by falling bricks and timbers, some head injury, and some orthopedic injury.(6) If one could ever know the extent and number of such injuries associated with a number of past earthquakes in Guatemala, one might begin to approximate some of the specific requirements for their care, such as how many operating sets, how many surgeons and how much suture material, etc. Using such data, standardized operating protocols could be developed for assessment of the early emergency medical response needs for use both within the stricken country and as a guide for the earliest international medical aid response. We clearly seem to need a mechanism for early determination of medical needs in a disaster situation, so that the required resources can be rapidly mobilized.

"EPIDEMIOLOGIC" MODEL FOR DISASTER RESEARCH

It is logical to suppose that a model might be useful for organizing the experience and information available in disaster research. A general epidemiologic or "natural history" model may be a useful start.

The time-line associated with disasters would fit the natural history model, in that there would be a period of primary intervention in which precautionary and preparedness measures may be taken, before the disaster strikes. These would be related to the expected agents, host populations (the potential victims), and environmental factors (including technological and cultural factors and resources for coping with disasters). These factors would relate specifically to given settings and the expectations or likelihood of certain types of disaster. In such potential events as floods, fires, toxic spills, etc., measures could also be taken to avert such disasters. Measures that may be taken at these stages can then be specified.

Secondary intervention includes early warning and prompt measures to lessen the potential impact of the disaster situations. This too would be related to the specific types of disaster and the settings in which they occur. Evacuation may be a key measure in this period. The need for and utility of measures of this type and the possibility of local, regional, national, and international aid may then be addressed.

With the occurrence of a disaster and its progression to full impact, the tertiary intervention stage comes into play. This includes identification of casualties and bringing these persons to health and medical services or bringing the resources to the location of the casualties (triage, transportation, treatment, and all the necessary communications and movement of personnel and supplies).

In addition, after the climax of the disaster, considerations for follow-up would be important for a number of reasons: prospective medical care, such as health protection through vaccination, safe food and water supply, restructuring and resupplying medical care facilities, assurance of adequate personnel, and other measures to maintain the benefits of the services applied at the height of the disaster. It would also be important, at this stage, to consider the ongoing emotional and psychological needs of the population that experiences the disaster and those who came to their aid.

A model of this sort would allow the proper placement of the available information, in order to construct a pattern from which generalizations may be developed. It would also allow the drawing of conclusions and lessons for future preparedness and disaster care in other settings This model is presented in outline form in Table III.

To carry the epidemiological model further, I propose that disasters be viewed in a rather classical epidemiological model in terms of the major factors that influence the incidence of a disease: agent factors, host factors, and environmental factors (Figure 1). In the matter of identifying agents and host factors, I am conducting a literature review for case reports regarding disasters that occurred in this decade. We are seeking such data as the type of disaster, date, location, number and type of casualties, setting, cultural and technological factors. In addition, we are contacting state, local and federal agencies in the United States for similar data and will acquire such data and specific reports as they are available from the North Atlantic Treaty Organization, International Red Cross, and the Pan American Health Organization. I am also collecting existing plans that have been devised by local and state governments.

Using this model, the agent is seen as the destructive event and the time over which it occurs. These features encompass the first and second components of the operational definition of disaster outlined above. The environment reflects the setting and the resources available and the host represents population and the number of casualties, usually occurring within a short period of time. The overall time phases listed according to a natural history model includes, as stated above, the stage of primary intervention (pre-disaster phase); secondary intervention (warning phase and imminent phase); tertiary intervention - early (impact phase, assessment phase, and initial aid phase); and tertiary intervention - late (reparative phase and recovery phase). The focus of the final report will be mainly the early tertiary intervention phase, including the assessment phase and the initial aid phase.

RESEARCH ABOUT DISASTER PREPAREDNESS

The "best" research to date about the consequences of disasters seems to have been conducted by sociologists such as Quarentelli, et al., at the Disaster Research Center (formerly located at the Ohio State University and now relocated to the University of Delaware). One of the major conclusions is that there are qualitative differences between everyday emergency medical services (EMS) and disaster emergency medical services.

The informative monograph, "Delivery of Emergency Medical Services in Disaster: Assumptions and Realities,"(7) explores the assumption commonly held in the United States that disaster emergency medical services are primarily an extension of everyday emergency medical services (EMS). Careful analysis of 33 real or simulated disasters in the United States that occurred during the mid-1970's revealed that there are indeed qualitative differences between everyday EMS and disaster EMS. In many instances the day-to-day system failed, not because it was disrupted by the disaster, but because of deficiencies inherent in the system: problems of communication, coordination, traffic control; and organization of medical services, lack of planning for medical decision-making in search and rescue or treatment efforts at the scene, inaccurate methods for estimating casualties, inadequate triage of casualties, poor record-keeping, inadequate measures for managing the "walking wounded" who arrive at the hospital and integration of new agencies, services and individuals into the overall response. Several of these problems were addressed in the U.S. National Disaster Exercise conducted in July of 1986 where the NATO Pilot Study Group participated as observers.

Texts that attempt to provide useful clinical information to practitioners about "disaster medicine," such as that written by Burkle, et al.,(8) draw heavily on military procedures that have been or could be used in civilian disasters, but cannot provide a useful guide to international participation in medical aspects of disaster preparedness because they too lack data about specific inquiries and illnesses encountered in civilian disasters. Texts that attempt to teach triage must similarly rely heavily on procedures and classification designed by the military for combat use.(9) The need to evaluate the interface between existing emergency medical services systems and the disaster medical response system has been identified as an important area of study in previous meetings of the pilot study group.

Some of the literature does contain some data useful in medical planning, such as that contained in PAHO reports and others about numbers and types of casualties associated with specific types of disaster. Several illustrative disaster reports currently being analyzed are included in the Bibliography of Specific Case Reports Section of this report.

As will be stated toward the end of this preliminary report, part of the completion of this project will require close inspection of data not generally available in the literature for estimation of injuries and illnesses associated with disasters.

INTERNATIONAL MEDICAL RESPONSE SYSTEMS: A PRIORITY FOR DISASTER RESEARCH

A recent presentation pointed to the need for research in international systems for medical response to disaster.(10) Drabek studied more than 1,000 publications regarding natural and man-made disasters. He studied eight disaster phases: planning, warning, evacuation, medical response, restoration, reconstruction; and two mitigating factors, hazard perceptions and adjustments. These factors were cross-tabulated with six levels of human social systems ranging in complexity from the micro system (individuals and groups) to macro systems (international systems). He identified both areas of previous research concentration and research gap. He found that the area of emergency medical response has been studied comparatively well on the individual and group level, but not on the level of international systems. Most research regarding international response focuses rather on the reconstruction phase as one might perhaps intuitively suspect. He concluded his presentation with the recommendation that we intensively pursue investigation into cross societal and international system responses during the emergency response period. His conclusion is certainly in concert with that of the NATO pilot study group meeting in Washington during the U.S. National Disaster Exercise held in July, 1986. The members emphasized that widespread human injury caused by the major chemical, earthquake, and radiation disasters of the recent past underscore the importance of research about emergency medical response in such situations. Ongoing study is critical since the risks of reoccurrence seem so great.

PLANS FOR CONTINUATION OF THE STUDY

The major objective of the next phase of study will be an intensive effort to collect data regarding specific injury and illness associated with specific disasters, and to look for some parameters useful for relating casualty volume to character or physical magnitude of the disaster. Based on such data I will try to outline components of the emergency medical response essential for an optimum overall disaster response effort. Such components include medical supplies, types and number of personnel, medical equipment, and hospital resources.

An effort will be directed to analysis of the written disaster plans for the fifty United States and the NATO countries to which I have access for information regarding existing capabilities and procedures for managing the health and medical aspects of disaster in a specific region with the hope of identifying strengths and weaknesses of the plan that depend on the type of disaster encountered. A plan may appear to be extremely well-suited to treatment of casualties sustained in earthquake, for example, but rather poorly suited for treatment of victims exposed to toxic chemicals or radiation.

An effort will be made to present the case for organization of international medical aid through planned medical response according to the type of disaster reported; sorting, and organization of supplies; and standardization of response procedures, such as standardized terms of reference, specific indications for expert assistance, and itemized equipment and supply rosters that can be used as a "checklist" in determining international aid deliveries.

While the effort may seem ambitious, I think it is the most proper place to begin systematic study of our medical response to casualties of many kinds of disaster in all parts of the world.

TABLE I

Types of Disasters

Natural	Man-Made
1. Tornado	1. Airplane crash
2. Hurricane	2. Building collapse
3. Tidal wave	3. Dam collapse
4. Flood	4. Explosion
5. Avalanche	5. Highway accident
6. Volcanic eruption	6. Mine disaster
7. Earthquake	7. Nuclear rector accident
8. Fire	8. Railroad wreck
	9. Panic crush
	10. Chemical spill
	11. Terrorist attack
	12. Disaster of sea

Famines and epidemics sometimes result from natural, man-made or a combination of the two.

Table II

Types of Resources

Medical	Non-Medical
Hospitals	Transportation system - land/highway use patterns
Emergency Medical Systems	Communication system
Personnel (physicians/nurses)	Food storage and distribution
Supplies/equipment/medicine	Public utilities
Paramedical units	Fire/police departments
	Buildings/shelters

TABLE III

I. Primary intervention

Preventative - precautionary and preparatory measures taken before a disaster strikes in order to minimize the destructive force of the agent and maximize the resistance and resiliency of the host and environment.

A. Predisaster phase

1. Environmental management, land treatment, reforestation, erosion control, coastal zone management, knowledge of historical patterns of disaster in each area, etc.

2. Vulnerability analysis

Collecting and assessing data on the endangered population and structures: including information on size, geographic distribution and general health and education status of population, structural integrity of buildings and lifeline systems, existing health, communication and transportation systems, and information regarding the performance of the above in previous disasters.

3. Preparedness analysis

Knowledge of standing disaster plans in different disaster prone areas, including operational capabilities to carry out such plans, emergency facilities, personnel and equipment, etc.

II. Secondary intervention

Preimpact - measures taken to warn of impending disaster and to lessen its destructive force if possible.

A. Warning phase

1. Hazard analysis.

Climatological studies, seismographic monitoring programs, etc.

2. Forecasting of specific hazards.

III. Tertiary intervention - early

Impact - Identification of needs and resources to meet those needs.

A. Impact phase - no intervention possible during this phase - except chaos.

B. Assessment phase

1. Identify the nature and cause of the emergency of disaster.

2. Determine immediate damage (e.g., number and types of casualties, damage to housing, public utilities, infrastructure, etc.).

3. Identify needs resulting from damage (e.g., treatment of injuries, provision of shelter/water, etc.).

C. Initial aid phase

1. Extrication

2. Initial aid at scene - triage, early treatment with appropriate flow of personnel and supplies via adequate transportation/communications.

3. Transportation from scene.

4. Initial aid at hospital or other facility receiving casualties.

IV. Tertiary intervention - late

Post impact - evaluate ongoing needs, rebuilding and future preparedness plans.

A. Reparative phase

1. Gather information for improving future disaster management.

2. Improve future preparedness plans - locally and in other disaster prone areas.

Agent	Destructive force
	The disaster event
	Time over which disaster occurs
Environment	Disaster Preplanning
	Available resources
Host	Casualties

Figure 1.

Figure 1. Five major components of a disaster include: destructive force, the event itself, resources available to deal with the consequences, the casualties and the time over which the damage occurs. These can be analyzed in an epidemiologic model as shown here.

Primary intervention	1. Predisaster phase
Secondary intervention	2. Warning phase
	3. Imminent phase
Tertiary intervention - early	4. Impact phase
	*5. Assessment phase
	*6. Initial aid phase
Tertiary intervention - late	7. Reparative phase
	8. Recovery phase

Figure 2.

*Major areas of emphasis for medical assistance following disaster.

Figure 2. Time phases of a disaster within a natural history model. The assessment phase and initial aid phase are the areas of major concentration for discussion about medical aspects of disaster preparedness.

REFERENCES

1. Rutherford WH, et al: The definition and classification of disasters. Injury, 15(1):10-2, 1983.

2. Irey NS: Environmental emergencies: their characteristics and variations. Milit Med, 150(4):191-9, 1985.

3. Parrish, et al: Epidemiology in public health planning for natural disasters. Public Health Reports (79)10:863-869, 1966.

4. Rutherford WH (Chairman): Report of the International Working Party on Disaster Medicine, 1980, London International Trauma Foundation.

5. Rutherford WH, et al: The definition and classification of disasters, Injury 15(1): 10-2, 1983.

6. Deville de Goyet C, et al: Earthquake in Guatemala: epidemiologic evaluation of the relief effort. PAHO Bulletin, Vol. 10-2, pp 95-109, 1976.

7. Quarantelli EL: Delivery of emergency medical services in Disasters: assumptions and realities. Irvington Publishers, Inc., New York, 1983.

8. Burkle F, Sanor P, Wolcott BW: Disaster Medicine, Medical Examination Publishing Co., Inc., New Hyde Park, NY, 1984.

9. Rund DA and Rausch TS: Triage, C.V. Mosby Co., St. Louis, 1981.

10. Drubeck E: The Disaster Research Legacy: Trends of a Decade, presented to the American Public Health Association, Washington DC, 1985.

BIBLIOGRAPHY OF SPECIFIC CASE REPORTS

EVENT CLASSIFICATION: MAN-MADE VS NATURAL

I. Man-Made Disasters

A. Train Disaster

1. The Kurunegula train disaster. Wijesekera C, et al: Ceyl Med J 1981, September; 26(3): 116-20.

2. The Nuneaton derailment. Miller PJ: Injury 1980, September; 12(2): 130-138.

3. The role of county hospital in a major disaster. Mallow Hospital and the Brittevant rail crash. Gaffney PR, et al: Ir Med J 1981, September; 74(9) 260-261.

4. Medical report on casualties in the Hokuriku Tunnel Train Fire in Japan with special reference to smoke-gas poisoning. Kutsumi A, et al: Mt. Sinai J Med (NY) 1979, September-October; 46(5): 469-474.

B. Chemical Disasters

1. Kepone: A chemical disaster in Hopewell, Virginia. Reich MR, et al: Int J Health Serv 1983; 13(2): 227-246 (60 ref.).

2. An eyewitness in Bhopal. Sutcliffe M: Br Med J (Clin Res) 1985, June 22; 290 (6485): 1883-1884.

3. Dioxin: Lessons from the Missouri experience. Bull Environ Contam Toxicol 1984, December; 33(6) 631-734.

4. Toxic gas: Pesticide plant leak wreaks disaster in India [news] Jayaraman KS: Nature 1984, December 13-19; 312 (5995): 581.

C. Airport Disaster

1. Experiences in medical coverage of airport disasters at Logan International Airport in Boston. Dudani N.: Aviat Space Environ Med 1985, May; 56(5): 457-461.

2. The Cincinnati DC-9 experience: lessons in aircraft and airport safety. Pane GA, et al: Aviat Space Environ Med 1985, May; 56(5) 457-461.

3. Mobilization of trauma teams for aircraft disasters. Star LD. et al: Aviat Space Environ Med 1980, November; 51(11) 1262-1266.

4. Medical coordination in airport disasters. Webb AC: Aviat Space Environ Med 1980, November; 51(11): 1256-1258.

5. A Metropolitan airport disaster plan - coordination of a multihospital response to provide on-site resuscitation and stabilization before evacuation. Dove DB, et al: J Trauma 1982, July;22(7): 550-559.

D. Ship Disasters

1. Disaster at sea: problem and prospects. Duffy JC: Milit Med 1979, September; 144(9): 616-618.

2. Activity of the medical profession on the occasion of a disaster at sea. The tragedy of the sinking of the Andrea Doria witnessed by the ship's doctor. Tortori-Donati B: J R Nov Med Serv 1980, spring; 66(1): 63-70.

E. Technological/Industrial Accidents

1. Responding to industrial accidents requires development of disaster plan. Star IM, et al: Occup Health Saf 1985, November; 55(11): 12-17.

2. Technological disasters in the Americas: A public health challenge. Wasserman E: WHO Chron 1985;, 39(3): 95-97.

F. Building Collapse

1. The Hyatt Regency skywalk collapse: an EMS-based disaster response. Orr SM, et al: Ann Emerg Med 1983, October; 12(10) 601-605.

G. Bus Accident

1. Autopsy of a disaster: the Martinez bus accident. Lewis FR, et al: J Trauma 1980, October; 20(10): 861-866.

H. Explosions

1. Terrorist bomb explosion in Bologna, Italy, 1980: an analysis of the effects and injuries sustained. Brismar B, et al: J Trauma 1982, March; 22(3) 216-220.

I. Nuclear/Radiation Accidents

1. The medical consequences of radiation accidents and nuclear war. Health Policy Committee, American College of Physicians. Ann Intern Med 1982, September; 97(3): 447-450.

II. Natural Disasters

A. Earthquakes

1. Postseismic reactions. Observations on a group of patients displayed psychic disorders determined by March 4, 1977 earthquake in Romania. Predescu V, et al: Neurol Psychiatr (Bucur) 1979, July-September; 17(3): 179-188.

2. Psychic manifestations in 117 young women of Bruharest after March 4, 1977 earthquake. Costa D, et al: Neurol Psychiatr (Bucur) 1981, January-March; 19(1): 45-51.

3. Disease epidemiology and earthquake disaster. The example of Southern Italy after the 23 November 1980 earthquake. Alexander D: Soc Sci Med 1981; 16(22): 1959-1969.

4. The 1980 earthquake in Southern Italy: rescue of trapped victims and mortality. de Bruycker M, et al: Bull WHO 1983; 61(6): 1021-1025.

5. Compressive eye injuries caused by earthquake. Cai YS, et al: Chin Med J [Engl] 1983, October; 96(10): 73-76.

6. Medical Consequences of the earthquake of 1886 in Charleston, South Carolina. Fitzgerald RH Jr.: South Med J 1985, April; 78(4): 458-462.

7. The 1980 earthquake in Southern Italy - morbidity and mortality. de Bruycker M, et al: Int J Epidemiol 1985, March; 14(1): 113-117.

8. Psychological stress and fatal heart attack: the Athens (1981) earthquake natural experiment. Trichopoulas D, et al: Lancet 1983, February; 1(8322): 441-444.

B. Fire

1. Treatment of burns casualties after fire at Bradford City football ground. Sharpe Dt, et al: Br Med J (Clin Res) 1985, October 5; 291(6500): 945-948.

2. Fire on the unit. Tousley MM: J Psychosoc Nurs Ment Health Serv 1985, August; 23(8): 6-9.

3. F-I-R-E! Evacuating St. Joseph's. Scanlon J: Dimens Health Serv 1983, May; 60(5): 18-19.

4. The MGM Grand Hotel fire: lessons learned from a major disaster. Buerk CA, et al: Arch Surg 1982, May; 117(5): 641-644.

5. Medical aspects of the 'Ash Wednesday bushfires'. Bacon AK: Aust Fam Physician 1983, December; 12(12): 838-839.

6. Management of mass burn casualties in a hospital with a burn unit. Keag J: Med J Aust 1980, April; 1(7): 303-305.

C. Floods

1. The Big Thompson Flood. Charney M, et al: Am J Forensic Med Pathol 1980, June; 1(2): 139-144.

2. Leads from the MMWR. Floods and immunization, United States-1983. JAMA 1983, May 6; 249(17): 2301.

3. Flood disasters and immunization--California. MMWR 1983, April 8; 32(13): 171-172, 178.

4. The Laingsburg flood disaster. Mac Mahon AG, et al: S Afr Med J 1983, May 289; (63(22): 865-866.

5. Gander flood spurs an emergency evacuation. Walsh C: Dimens Health Serv 1984, January; L1(1): 30-31.

6. Mortality from flash floods: A review of national weather service reports, 1969-1981. French J, et al: Public Health Rep 1983, November-December; 98(6): 584-588.

7. Increased leukemia, lymphoma, and spontaneous abortion in Western New York following a flood disaster. Janerick DT, et al: Public Health Rep 1981, July-August; 96(4): 350-356.

D. Hurricanes

1. Hurricanes and hospital emergency-room visits--Mississippi, Rhode Island, Connecticut. MMWR 1986, January 3; 34(51-52): 765-770.

2. Gulf Coast hospitals withstand Hurricane Frederic's barrage [news]. Friedman E: Hospitals 1979, October 16; 53(20): 17-18.

3. Emotional and physical distress following Hurricane Agnes in Wyoming Valley of Pennsylvania. Logue JN, et al: Public Health Rep 1979, November-December; 94(6): 495-502.

4. Cyclone '78 in Sri Lanka--the mental health trial. Patrick V, et al: Br J Psychiatry 1981, March; 138:210-216.

5. Morbidity of Hurricane Frederic. Longmire AW, et al: Ann Emerg Med 1984, May; 13(5): 334-338.

6. Multiple casualties caused by a gale. Illingsworth RN, et al: Arch Emerg Med 1984, March; 1(1): 57-60.

7. Psychotic reactions to a natural disaster: Hurricane Alicia. Carlson RJ, et al: Tex Med 1985, July; 81(7):48-49.

E. Tornado

1. Tornado disaster--North Carolina, South Carolina, March 28, 1984. MMWR 1985, April 19; 34(15): 205-206, 211-213.

2. The December 2, 1982 tornado of Saline and Pulaski counties: implications for injury prevention. Leibovich M: J Arkansas Med Soc 1983, July; 80(2): 98-102.

3. Emotional effects of the Omaha tornado. Rosenberg SA, et al: Nebr Med J 1980, February; 65(2): 24-26.

F. SNOW

1. Blizzard morbidity and mortality: Rhode Island, 1978. Faich G, et al: Am J Public Health 1979, October; 69(10): 1050--1052.

2. Health consequences of the snow disaster in Massachusetts, February 6, 1978. Geass RI, et al: Am J Public Health 1979, October; 69(10): 1047-1049.

3. Public health impact of a snow disaster. MMWR 1982, December 31; 31(51): 695-696.

G. Volcano

1. Deaths during the May 18, 1980 eruption of Mount St. Helens. Eisele JW, et al: N Engl J Med 1981, October 15; 305(16): 931-936.

2. Death by volcano. NZ Med J 1982, February 24; 95(702): 115-116.

3. Acute effects of volcanic ash from Mt. St. Helens on lung function in children. Buist AS, et al: Am Rev Respir Dis 1983, June; 127(6): 714-719.

4. Mount St. Helens eruptions: the acute respiratory effects of volcanic ash in a North American community. Baxter PJ, et al: Arch Environ Health 1983, May-June; 38(3): 138-143.

5. Ocular effects following the volcanic eruptions of Mount St. Helens. Fraunfelder FT, et al: Arch Ophtholmal 1983, March; 101(3): 376-378.

6. Mount St. Helens eruptions, May 18 to June 12, 1980. An overview of the acute health impact. Baxter PJ, et al: JAMA 1981, December 4; 246(22): 2585-2589.

H. Miscellaneous

1. Major disasters. The patient with multiple injuries. Evans RF. Br J Hosp Med 1979, October; 22(4): 329-332.

2. Catastrophes et morts collectives. Recent American experiences in mass deaths. Eckert WG: Am J Forensic Med Pathol 1980, March; 1(1): 77-79.

3. Care of eye injuries in disasters [editorial]. Mallek D: Can J Ophthalmol 1980, July; 15(3):109-110.

4. Research issues and directions in the epidemiology of health effects of disasters. Logue JN, et al: Epidemiol Rev 1981; 31: 140-162.

5. Mass casualties: a seminar. Med J Zambia 1979, December1980 January; 14(1):1-17.

6. Catastrophic accidents - a 40 year review. Stat Bull Metrop Life Found 1982, April-June; 63(2):2-5.

7. Some health consequences of a natural disaster. Clayer JR, et al: Med J Aust 1985, September 2; 143(5):182-184.

8. Organization of hospital medical care of mass casualties in peace time disasters. Weiss DB, et al: Int Surg 1982, October-December; 67(4 Suppl):400-402.

FUNCTUONAL RESPONSIBILITIES OF EMERGENCY DEPARTMENT ATTENDING PHYSICIAN

[The Senior Attending Physician in the Emergency Department is in charge of all activities occurring in the Emergency Department. The following are his/her specific responsibilities during a disaster situation.]

1) Determine type of disaster, location of disaster, approximate number of major and minor injuries to be triaged to OSU, and estimated time of arrival.

2) Activate the hospital disaster plan by notifying the administrator on call to the E.D. and the hospital page operator. In addition, notify the page operator which services need to report to physicians' pool. (Examples: Casualties from a tornado strike will require large numbers of residents and attendants from general surgery, orthopedics, and neurosurgery. Casualties from an explosion and fire will require residents and attendants from general and plastic surgery. Casualties from a mass food poisoning will require physicians from internal medicine.)

3) Determine if a Triage Team is needed at the disaster site and designate the Triage Team. Triage Team consists of Emergency Medicine attending and/or senior emergency resident and/or 3rd,/4th/5th year surgical resident, and Emergency Department nurse.

4) Assign a physician (3rd-year E.M. resident, or 3rd/4th/5th-year surgery resident) to function as the Triage Physician.

5) Direct Emergency Department clerk to initiate Emergency Department physicians call list.

6) Discharge all non-emergency patients from Emergency Department.

7) Assign general surgery, emergency medicine, internal medicine, and specialty service physicians to treatment care area.

8) Ensure that all disaster patients are triaged to the appropriate patient care area.

9) Do not provide direct patient care. Rather, prioritize patient care. Determine which patients should go to x-ray, surgery, etc. Maintain patient flow by seeing that patients are transferred expeditiously to operating rooms, intensive care units, secondary triage areas, etc. Ensure that only essential x-rays and other diagnostic studies are performed in the Emergency Department.

10) Ensure that all patients have adequate medical and nursing care. Notify physician pool whenever additional physicians are needed. Notify Charge Nurse regarding need for additional supplies and personnel.

11) Maintain contact with disaster scene and determine number of additional casualties to be triaged to OSU.

12) Maintain contact with Disaster Control Center and provide updates on casualties expected, casualties received, personnel requirements, etc.

RESPONSIBILITIES OF CASUALTY PHYSICIAN*

1) Identify yourself to the Emergency Department Attending Physician. He/she will assign you to a location where you will provide care to patients as they arrive.

2) There will be nurses assigned to each Emergency Department area who will help with patient care. Identify yourself to the nurse assigned to your area.

3) In a disaster, patients must be evaluated, stabilized and transferred as quickly as possible to the O.R., ICU, 2° triage areas, etc.

4) Do not order laboratory tests or x-rays which are not necessary for immediate patient management.

5) The Emergency Department Attending Physician will have ultimate authority regarding patient management and disposition decisions.

6) When you have determined that a patient is ready for the O.R., ICU, etc., inform the Charge Nurse.

7) Do not leave the Emergency Department until you are dismissed by the Emergency Department Attending Physician.

* EM, surgical, Internal Medicine, or speciality service residents and faculty.

RESPONSIBILITIES OF TRIAGE PHYSICIAN*

1) Report to triage area.

2) Put on identification vest.

3) Identify self to Triage Nurse and Triage Clerk.

4) Work with Triage Nurse to ensure that triage area has adequate transport personnel, wheelchairs, and gurneys. If not, notify Charge Nurse.

5) Meet and briefly examine patients arriving to the Emergency Department and triage according to the following criteria:

Red tag - Critical Care (immediately life-threatening)

a) Triage to Trauma I or "shock-trauma"

Orange tag - Serious Major Injury (potentially, though not immediate life-threatening)

a) Triage to surgery treatment area

Yellow tag - Stable injury

a) Triage to medicine treatment area

Blue tag - First Aid

a) Triage to Observation and other East Corridor rooms

Black tag - DOA

a) Triage to exam room 4.

b) Do not attempt resuscitation.

6) Communicate patient destination to Triage Clerk, patient escort, and write on disaster tag.

7) Continue triage until you have been notified by Emergency Department Attending Physician that no more patients will be arriving. You will then be assigned to a patient treatment area.

NOTE: Your job is to triage, not to treat patients. Move patients from the triage area expeditiously. You should spend no more than one to two minutes with each patient.

* Triage Physician is a 3rd-year EM resident, EM Faculty, or 3rd/4th or 5th-year surgery resident as assigned by Attending Emergency Department Physician.

EMERGENCY DEPARTMENT DISASTER PLAN

Table of Contents

V. Functional Responsibilities

A. Emergency Department Attending Physician

B. Casualty Physician

C. Triage Physician

D. Charge Nurse

E. Emergency Department Nursing Staff

F. Emergency Department Clerical Staff

VI. Use of the Disaster Call List

VII. Miscellaneous Guidelines

Purpose: This plan is developed as a guide and reference for Emergency Department response to disasters of any kind.

Verification of Disaster

Anyone within the Emergency Department who is informed of a major disaster will ascertain:

A. Estimated number of casualties, anticipated number of casualties to be received by University Hospital, and estimated time of arrival;

B. Cause of the disaster, e.g., food poisoning, tornado, explosion;

C. Location of disaster;

D. Name and phone number of the individual notifying the hospital.

The above information will be reported to the senior Administrator/ Coordinator on duty at the time.

Activation of Disaster Plan

The Attending Physician in the Emergency Department will determine when the Emergency Department no longer can handle emergency patients plus the anticipated number of casualties and will notify hospital administration accordingly.

Emergency Department Function

The Emergency Department will serve as the triage area. All disaster casualties will come to University Hospital via the Emergency Department. The function of the Emergency Department in a disaster is to provide primary and secondary triage of disaster victims.

I. Primary Triage

A. Primary triage will occur just inside the automatic doors near the first storage room.

B. Primary triage is staffed by the senior surgical resident on duty, an Emergency Department RN and an Emergency Department Clerk. Primary triage is staffed by attending ED physician until he/she is relieved by the senior surgical resident.

C. The function of primary triage is:

1. Initial triage of victim into secondary triage areas within the Emergency Department;

2. Initial numbering and tagging of disaster victims;

3. Keeping a log that identifies, by number, dispersion of disaster victim;

D. Numbered charts with correspondingly numbered valuables envelopes and bracelets are placed on each disaster victim at primary triage.

E. Patients are triaged according to the severity of their injuries into the following secondary triage areas:

1. Critical care	-Trauma Room I and Shock Trauma
2. Serious major injury/illness	-Surgery Treatment Area
3. Stable injury/illness	-Medicine Treatment Area
4. First Aid	-Observation Room S77 RH and East corridor as needed
5. DOA	-Rm S70 RH

II. Secondary Triage

A. The purpose of secondary triage is to provide more extensive patient assessment and treatment as the situation indicates;

B. Patients are transported from secondary triage to the appropriate place within the hospital.

FUNCTIONAL RESPONSIBILITIES OF THE CHARGE NURSE

I. A. The charge nurse on duty at the onset of a disaster will assume charge responsibilities until the head nurse arrives;

B. When the head nurse arrives he/she will assume charge nurse responsibilities;

C. If the head nurse cannot be reached and there is not an assistant head nurse in charge, the first assistant head nurse to arrive will assume charge nurse responsibilities;

II. Assign clerical staff to initiate:

A. Physician call list

B. Nursing call list

C. Clerical staff call list

III. Open disaster trunks that are stored in Trauma II

A. Move First Aid Trunk S-77 (Observation, East Corridor)

B. Move Triage Supply Trunk stored in S-73 to Triage Area

IV. A. Put on the red vest located in Triage Supply Trunk which identifies you as the charge person.

B. Make sure that the triage nurse and Emergency Department nurses in charge of the treatment areas are garbed in the blue vests located in Triage Supply Trunk. This identifies them as the person (nurse) of authority in that area.

V. Assign staff to:

A. Assist the Attending Emergency Physician in discharging as many patients as possible from the Emergency Department.

VI. Then reassign staff as necessary and according to the following directive:

A. Triageur should remain at triage (directly behind the double doors leading into the Emergency Department - beside the storeroom) to help the assigned physician with triage of disaster victims.

B. Assign an attendant to First Aide area (observation - East Corridor).

C. Assign nursing staff to treatment areas as the need dictates.

D. It is essential that the charge nurse only directs activity, i.e.,

1. remains free of patient care;

2. remains visible to all people (in front of main nursing station).

E. When additional help arrives assignments should be made as the need dictates.

VII. Communicates with disaster control center to request nursing personnel from nursing personnel pool as necessary.

FUNCTIONAL RESPONSIBILITY OF EMERGENCY DEPARTMENT NURSING STAFF

I. Staff on duty at the time of the disaster will be assigned to secondary triage areas within the Emergency Department. Emergency Department staff members will be given blue vests to wear for the purpose of identification. Emergency Department staff members will direct the necessary care and act as resource people for other staff members assigned initially to the Emergency Department.

II Emergency Department staff coming in from home will report to the charge nurse (wearing a red vest) for assignment.

Functional Responsibilities of the Emergency Department Clerical Staff

The supervisor will be notified immediately and she will initiate the call list. Everyone is to call the name under theirs. If that person is unavailable, go on to the next. If the supervisor is not available, the call list should be initiated by a clerical specialist as assigned by the charge nurse. Assignment of clerical staff will be done as additional staff arrive on the unit.

Use of Disaster Call List

I. In the case of a disaster, the disaster call lists will be initiated here in the Emergency Department.

II. When you receive a call that there is a disaster, you are to call the person below you on the call list. If the person below you cannot be reached, you should continue on down the list until you reach someone at home. It is therefore necessary to keep a disaster call list readily available to you at home.

MISCELLANEOUS GUIDELINES

I. If hospital and/or home communications are impossible for any reason, all Emergency Department staff are to report to duty.

II. Identification may be required.

III. Uniforms are preferred, but optional in a disaster situation . identification. Arm bands will be provided to staff not in uniform.

COMMON PSYCHOLOGICAL THEMES IN SOCIETIES' REACTION TO TERRORISM AND DISASTERS

John C. Duffy, M.D., FAPA, FAsMA

Assistant Surgeon General, U.S. Public Health Service
U.S.A.

INTRODUCTION

In this presentation I will outline the major components of disasters (man-made and natural) and terrorism. In each I will develop their common scenarios, dominant psychological themes, and impacts on society. We shall then explore the remarkable psychological similarities in terms of the human beings touched by these events; i.e., the universality of anxiety in such experiences and the long-term psychological price to be paid; i.e., the post-traumatic stress disorder (PTSD).

Let's begin our review with disasters. For all its importance and immediacy, the problem of natural disasters remains unsolved. On the one hand, it involves protecting man from nature; on the other hand, in light of observed ecological crisis, it frequently involves protecting nature from man. Excessive activity toward a more efficient use of nature and toward its reformation can lead to anthropogenic natural disasters.

As Beinin noted, "In his treatment of nature, in reevaluating his attitude to nature, and in his endeavor to reach 'infinita potestas,' man has become highly inventive, though not very wise." (1)

Since ancient times, man has observed the devastating and depressing effects of natural disasters. He struggles against them, always unsuccessfully. He has desperately contrived means of protection never effective enough. Passive acceptance of his lot always predominated over useful activity.

Natural disasters interfere with all spheres of life, suddenly bringing about drastic changes in routine for a certain period of time. They also cause considerable long-term damage and have public health and other unexpected consequences. A natural disaster lays bare the latent malfunctions of the public, state organizations, and governments. It also reveals the impulse of altruism, people's feelings of compassion, and their readiness to help each other.

It is interesting to speculate about the time that man first assumed responsibility for a disaster. When in the dim past did man differentiate those disasters that were "an act of God" from those for which he alone must accept responsibility? Certainly, the concept of "man-made disaster" has a chilling effect, with all its implications of culpability.

Health and Medical Aspects of Disaster Preparedness
Edited by J.C. Duffy
Plenum Press, New York, 1990

When nature lashes out, society takes a stoic view; the gods have acted, taking their mysterious toll. If, on the other hand, man's acts of commission or omission result in disaster, there is often a special quality of guilt and responsibility along with anger and non-acceptance, such manmade disasters carry a heavy burden in terms of chronic mental ill health.

I have chosen three man-made disasters that bring home the horror of such experiences. In each disaster the lives of hundreds of persons, their relatives or friends, and rescue workers are touched, leaving a psychic scar.

WALL OF WATER

On February 26, 1972, an enormous slag dam, the end product of mining operations of the Buffalo Mining Company, split apart. In the path of thousands of tons of water and black mud was Buffalo Creek Valley in West Virginia.

In the colorless words of the engineers, the water expended its force in no more than 15 minutes at any one point in the 18-mile-long valley. A more tragic description could be found among the muddy residue of human bodies, houses, trailers, cars, and other debris. The wall of water was to rush past towns whose names could not be found on any map--Lundale, Pardee, Becco, Crites, Saunders, all just below the dam, completely vanished.

In many respects, Buffalo Creek Valley was typical of the mining communities of the region. It had a total of five active mines, as well as ugly strip-mining: proud families with well cared for homes and a strong sense of community. Nearly all the residents depended upon the mines for their economic livelihood.

A team of investigators from the Department of Psychiatry, University of Cincinnati Medical Center, went to Buffalo Creek to assess the psychological damage. Headed by psychiatrist James L. Titchner, they found a definable clinical entity characterized by a well delineated group of clinical symptoms they labeled a "traumatic neurosis." (2)

Unlike the passive and accepted reactions to natural disasters, a group of 654 survivors from 160 families began a legal action against the Buffalo Mining Company. In 1974, the suit was settled for 13.5 million dollars. Of particular interest was the fact that 6 million was for psychological damages.

BALL OF FIRE

It is the Memorial Day weekend, 1977. A popular nightclub in Kentucky, with the unusual name Beverly Hills, was having an especially busy evening. Reportedly a "Land of Oz Complex," it was a maze of bars, dining rooms, and a cabaret room, all opulently decorated in a style William Randolph Hearst would have approved. Its main business was the catering of special dinners, wedding and retirement parties, and bar mitzvahs.

That night, there was every sort of gathering. It was in the Zebra Room that fire was to explode at 9:00 p.m. A full twenty minutes were to pass, while employees attempted to put out the fire. In what can only be described as denial, when the warning was finally announced, persons watching a comedy act in the cabaret section thought it was part of the script.

When the last ember was distinguished, there were 164 dead and 60 injured. Nearly two years later, evidence of mental trauma could still be found. Rescue workers, often seen as "immune" from stress because they are "professionals," indeed pay an emotional price. For example, a rescue worker developed a significant depressive reaction: her dreams were interrupted by the screams of trapped human beings in the club. A proud man, unable to explain the change in his personality after escaping the fire, thought it was not "manly" to seek psychiatric treatment.

COLLISION COURSE

The final disaster is one that is also man-made. It is unique in that it almost always involves strangers, without any supporting social systems and, in my judgment, is for the most part ignored in terms of mental health assistance.

On March 27, 1977, the name Tenerife, an obscure part of the Canary Island off the Coast of Africa, became both familiar and forever associated with terror. It was on a foggy runway on this semi-tropical island of Tenerife that two jumbo 747's collided. All 251 persons on board the KLM plane died; on the Pan American Airways plane, 326 passengers lost their lives, but 80 survived. Prior to Tenerife, there had been only two other fatal accidents involving 747's. In 1974, a Lufthansa 747 crashed on takeoff in Nairobi, Kenya, with 59 dead. In 1976, an Iranian Air Force 747 broke apart above Huete, Spain, killing 17.

When the KLM plane hit the PAN AM aircraft, it ripped off a huge piece of the top section of the fuselage. The pilot, Captain Grubbs, and co-pilot, Bragg, were dropped into the first class cabin below the flight deck. In some fashion, Captain Grubbs got to the ground, where he began beating it. A purser found him kneeling, rocking back and forth, and mumbling, "What have I done to these people?"

The scene was so chaotic and the bodies so distorted that 114 persons were never identified. They have been buried in a mass grave purchased by Pan American Airway in Orange County, California.

But unlike Buffalo Creek or Beverly Hills, there would be no investigative team of mental health specialists. In fact, typical of many commercial aircraft accidents, there was a denial of any need for crisis mental health intervention. And yet, the psychological response for the survivors of aircraft accidents is not that different, except for the absence of a strong "community" support system that is so typical in other disasters.

When disaster renders a community helpless within a society, that society responds by protecting its community from further loss of lives and property. In its own best interest, for the sake of social integrity, the society feels further obligated to salvage and restore the community structure to a viable form so its members can resume their productive roles and thereby restore the community as a functional part of the whole society. Over and beyond the physical damage to property, bodily injuries, and fatalities of citizens, there is another loss or drain on the community's resources. This drain is in the form of the negative effects of the emotional shock suffered by the bereft, and the incapacity of many individuals to resume employment due to the long-phase effects of stress, guilt, or other trauma related directly to the disaster.

STAGES AFTER A DISASTER

The **heroic phase** of a disaster occurs at the time of and immediately after the crisis. Emotions are strong and direct. Individuals are called upon to act to save their own lives, as well as the lives of others. The most important resources during this phase are family groups, neighbors, and emergency teams.

The **honeymoon phase** extends from one week to six months after a disaster. For those who have survived, even with loss of loved ones and possessions, there is a strong sense of having shared with others a dangerous, catastrophic experience and having lived through it. Various officials and governmental persons promise all kinds of help and the survivors anticipate that there will soon be considerable aid in solving their problems. Preexisting and emergency community groups, which develop from the specific needs of the disaster, are especially important community resources during this period.

The **disillusionment phase** lasts from two months to a year or more. Strong feelings of disappointment, anger, resentment, and bitterness may appear if delays or failures occur and the hopes for the promised aid are not fulfilled. Outside agencies may pull out and some of the indigenous community groups may weaken or become unadaptive. Also contributing to this stage may be the gradual loss of the feeling of "shared community" as the survivors concentrate on rebuilding their own lives and solving their individual problems.

And the last phase, **reconstruction**, occurs when the persons realize that they will need to solve their problems by themselves and gradually assume responsibility for doing so. During this phase, which generally lasts for several years following the disaster, the appearance of new buildings and the development of new programs and plans serve to reaffirm their belief in their community and in their own capabilities and abilities. When these are delayed, however, the emotional problems that appear may be serious and intense. Community groups with a long-term investment in the community and its people become key elements in this phase.

Let's summarize the important psychological stressors associated with disasters and their impact on the individual, that is, the victim.

In terms of response:
- 1/3 little stress
- 2/3 stress and mild depression
- 1% or less suffer severe impairment

The initial human reaction is:
- 12-15% "cool and collected"
- 75% temporarily stunned and bewildered

What are the severe stressors?
- Sudden loss of loved one(s)
- Severe disruption of life routine
- Sudden loss of basic security needs; e.g., home, food, supply
- Possible sense of loss from bodily injury

Symptoms during civilian disasters:
- Acute grief
- Severe anxiety/panic reactions
- Both of the above may approach or assume transient psychotic or psychotic-like behavior that would warrant the diagnosis of brief, reactive psychoses.

The disaster syndrome is present in up to 75% of victims during the impact phase. It includes: absence of emotion, inhibition of activity, docility, indecision, lack of responsiveness, automatic behavior, and physiological manifestation of fear.

We now turn to the subject of terrorism. There is, of course, no anatomy, psychologically speaking, of the "disaster" itself. Here the disaster is man-made, uniquely, in that the disaster is crafted by men. The victim is, as always, the recipient of psychological damage. There is an aspect of the victims of terrorism which makes their plight so much worse. The man-made disaster victims realize a finite conclusion and expect relief. For the terrorist victim there is no end in sight, and no expected relief. However, in terrorism we do indeed have a unique psychological anatomy, namely, the terrorists. Who are they? Is there a logic behind their acts?

Some experts argue that political terrorists are driven to commit acts of violence as a consequence of psychological forces, and that their special psycho-logic is constructed to rationalize acts they are psychologically compelled to commit. Thus, the principal argument is that individuals are drawn to the path of terrorism in order to commit acts of violence, and their special logic, which is grounded in their psychology and reflected in their rhetoric, becomes the justification for their violent acts.

Considering the diversity of causes to which terrorists are committed, the uniformity of their rhetoric is striking. Polarizing and absolutist, it is a rhetoric of "us versus them." It is a rhetoric without nuance, without shades of gray. "They," the establishment, are the source of all evil in vivid contrast to "us," the freedom fighters, consumed by righteous rage. And, if "they" are the source of our problems, it follows inevitably, in the special psycho-logic of the terrorist, that "they" must be destroyed. It is the only just and moral thing to do. Once one accepts the basic premises, the logical reasoning is flawless. Shall we then conclude because their reasoning is so logical that terrorists are psychologically well balanced and that terrorist campaigns are the product of a rationally derived strategic choice?

There is, of course, no necessary relationship between emotional health and logic. Some delightfully happy and psychologically well balanced individuals are utterly unable to track their way through a syllogism. And the tight logical structure of the well organized paranoid is a marvel to behold. In a jewel of a treatise, the mathematical psychologist von Domarus has delineated the logical structure of delusions, a logic which he has named "paralogical." (3) The fixed logical conclusion of the terrorist, that the establishment must be destroyed, is driven by the terrorist's search for identity, and that as he strikes out against the establishment, he is attempting to destroy the enemy within.

Our interest, however, in this presentation is with victims. Unlike our disaster victims, we define the terrorist victim as a hostage.

What is government's responsibility and how do the victim views them? In the terrorist/hostage scenario, government is also tested--not for relief, but for its ability to respond to collective bargaining.

It has been known for some time that hostages represent the power to hurt in its purest form. Terrorists choose this strategy in order to manipulate a government's political decisions. For purposes of analysis, it is assumed that terrorists genuinely seek the concessions they demand. Their preference is for government compliance rather than for resistance.

Terrorist bargaining is essentially a form of blackmail or extortion. Terrorists seize hostages in order to affect a government's choices, which are controlled both by expectations of outcome (what the terrorists are likely to do given a specific government reaction) and preferences (such as humanitarian values).

Each terrorist episode is actually a round in a series of games between government and terrorist. And worse, potential victims know the game.

Terrorists may also affect the structure of the government's decision by promising rewards for compliance. Recalling that terrorism represents an iterative game, the release of hostages unharmed when ransom is paid underwrites a promise in the future. Sequential release is also a method of making a promise credible. Terrorists may also try to make their demands appear legitimate, not only so that governments may appear to satisfy popular grievances rather than the whims of terrorists, but also to attempt to convince the victims that their cause is just. Hence terrorists may ask that food be distributed to the poor, for example. Terrorists may also try to delink their case from that of other terrorists, to convince governments that giving in, in this instance, will not affect their position vis-a-vis other terrorists. Rewarding compliance is not easy to reconcile with making threats credible. For example, if terrorists use publicity to emphasize their threat to kill hostages (which they frequently do), they may also increase the costs of compliance for the government because of the attention they have attracted. The result for the hostage victim is confusion and is often resolved by identification with the aggressor.

In considering the payoffs for each side, one must also take into account the costs associated with the bargaining process. The longer the hostage crisis drags on, the greater the costs to all players--terrorist, government, and victim. The question is who loses most and thus is more likely to concede. Each wishes to make delay more costly to the other.

The resolution to this is bargaining. Most importantly, bargaining depends on the existence of a common interest between two parties. It is unclear, particularly to the victims, whether their lives are a sufficient common interest to insure a compromise outcome that is preferable to no agreement for both sides.

Armed rescue attempts are another effort to break the bargaining stalemate.

Let's summarize the common features which the victims of disasters and terrorism experience. Both experience an unpredictable disruption of their lives; they are in a helpless position as bargaining chits between government and local authorities or terrorists; they experience grief and loss of freedom and threats to their bodily integrity and, ultimately, their life.

Centers have been established to deal with victims of hostage situations. They also specialize in the treatment of individuals who have experienced torture. The experience of these treatment centers is a high degree of symptomology in both groups. This past September in Paris, the Third International Conference of Centers Assisting Victims of Organized Violence addressed the common psychological themes of these patients and treatment strategies. Among their treatment goals are:

1. To link the trauma with the symptom.
2. To encourage an understanding of their symptoms in light of their previous experience and culture background.
3. To help the victims regain control of their lives; to reestablish a sense of personal safety in daily living.

Let's look at clinical issues. We have reviewed "response" to disasters and terrorism. I suggest that while we tend to compartmentalize these experiences, suggesting different psychological themes or issues, in fact they are psychologically closely related in etiology, treatment, and outcome. Let's review these common aspects, and my major thesis which is: that the common denominator for all of these experiences is the post-traumatic stress disorder (PTSD), the result of a loss of sense of personal safety.

The concept of post-traumatic stress disorder has a long history in both military and civilian medicine, but formal recognition and diagnostic criteria have only recently been given. Post-traumatic stress disorder is classed among the anxiety disorders. Yet, the diagnostic signs and symptoms required for this diagnosis include many features usually associated with depression. Markedly diminished interest in activities, detachment from others, constricted affect, guilt, impairment of memory and concentration, sleep difficulties, and recurrent thoughts of death.

Recent reviews of PTSD have noted that controversy continues to rage over the disorder. Are the symptoms evidence only of a consistent process set in motion following any major threat to one's security? Does the condition merit consideration as a clinical entity to be classified separately in our diagnostic scheme? Are the stress disorders merely variants of personality disorders? Is massive psychological trauma the etiologic agent? May the condition be induced in adulthood without preceding genetic and/or constitutional determinants or early traumatic experiences? In short, are the phenomena of the stress disorders only reflections of psychological processing of information signifying existential threat, or are they representative of other (possibly preceding) psychopathological and/or neural changes?

We have, then, a clinical condition induced by either a single, massive psychological assault or by recurrent or continued exposure to experiences associated with violent death, destruction, and/or mutilation of others, which induces high intensity emotional arousal. The emotions of fear, terror, and helpless despair are followed by a number of constant yet repetitive behavioral, cognitive, and physiological processes. In many, withdrawal from exposure, non-recurrence of exposure, or avoidance of memory-arousing experiences similar to the initial stressing events is followed by extinction of these phenomena. In some, the extinction is only partial; somatic arousal still may be observed when the gross clinical symptoms have remitted. Other patients go on to suffer delayed, recurrent, or persistent display of the consequences of the overwhelming emotional assault. I emphasize "emotional" and not "psychological." Emotions are a part of stimulus facilitation. Depending on the intensity of stimulation, it may facilitate or destroy cognitive processing. Among those who fail to recover from the initial assault are a group who suffer recurrent or persistent clinical symptoms and demonstrate evidence of a conditioned emotional response.

In summary, we have reviewed two severely traumatic experiences in society--man-made disasters and terrorism. We have also analyzed how the victims of terrorism share all the psychological elements characteristic of man-made disasters, and also how they share the same expression, psychologically speaking, the post-traumatic stress disorder.

Psychologically speaking, the disaster victim and the hostage victim share much in common.

REFERENCES

1. Beinin L: Medical Consequences of Natural Disasters. Berlin. Springer-Verlag, 1985.

2. Titchner JL, Kapp FT: Family and Character Change at Buffalo Creek. Am J Psychiatry 133: 295-299, 1976.

3. von Domarus E. The Specific Laws of Logic in Schizophrenia. In Kasanin JL (ed.) Language and Thought is Schizophrenia. New York. Norton, 1944, pp. 104-14.

PSYCHOLOGICAL TRAINING OF DISASTER WORKERS

F.C. ANTONINI, Ph.D.

Professor, University of Montreal
Montreal, Canada

SUMMARY

That catastrophic events may have a deep psychological impact on their victims seems almost too obvious to be questioned. The important and crippling sequelae observed after such episodes in the lives of some persons are no longer the object of controversy. They have now been identified as a well-defined pathological syndrome: the "post-traumatic stress disorder" (PTSD) (1).

However, it is only recently that psychological assistance and support for the victims of disastrous occurrences have been **effectively implemented.** In many, but unfortunately not all cases, they are a part of the emergency efforts (2,3).

A even less degree of attention has been given to the psychological trauma and stress undergone by the members of rescue teams; the impact and consequences on their health, personal lives and that of their families and that of their performance at work. I would like to address this particular problem, the reasons for its existence and the necessity to include a psychological preparation during the formal training of these workers and/or at least, include aftermath-disaster debriefing sessions in the organization of their duties.

I shall review briefly the concept of stress and human adaptation and will insist specifically on the stressing elements attached to disasters and their psychological effects on the rescuers. I will also give some practical information, suggestions and guidelines aiming at the better mental preparation of the relief workers.

I. STRESS AND THE STRESS RESPONSE

Stress is a widely used word and has undergone many changes in its meaning since it was first coined and developed independently by Cannon and Selye (4,5). As such, stress can be understood as the general and nonspecific organic response of an individual in the presence of what is called an element(s) of stress or "stressor" most generally coming from the environment.

Health and Medical Aspects of Disaster Preparedness
Edited by J.C. Duffy
Plenum Press, New York, 1990

The stress response presents three stages:

1) The **Alarm Reaction** during which the organism stimulated by the external or internal so-called stressor(s) mobilizes its nervous and muscular resources for intervention.

2) The **Adaptation Period** during which the individual acts in the situation using old or new strategies devised for a better coping. The Adaptation Period is normally followed by a period of more or less pronounced withdrawal and rest from the stressing agents during which the organism replenishes the energy used, and returns to its normal homeostasis. (previous equilibrium)

3) Whereas the two previous stages are normal, a third "the **Exhaustion Period**" can take place when the organism, unable to stop its activity, undergoes a rapid depletion of its resources leading to exhaustion. This occurs when the period of adaptation exceeds the usual capabilities of the organism, either because the strategies were not adequately contrived or the situation was requiring more effort and time than the individual could handle or both. Beyond a certain point, the period of exhaustion is irreversible and death ensues.

One can resist acute stress resulting from short duration exposure to only one stressing episode of significant magnitude, and to long-term chronic stress stemming from small but recurring incidents.

The first recorded and most famous example of acute stress is that of the first Marathon runner, the Greek soldier who died of exhaustion delivering his urgent message after a long and strenuous run for which he was not trained.

II. THE STRESSORS

Stressors are of a multiple nature. For example, the following are widely accepted as stressors: cold and heat exposure, strenuous muscular exercise, sleep deprivation, noise either unexpected or at high level or for long periods of time, fatigue, fasting, living in a crowded environment, etc. Also stressors are: physical illness, surgery, loss of significant other, social changes, social isolation. The list is long and for reasons which will be developed later, there is in fact no end to the lists of stressors. However, one tends to classify stressors into three categories:

1) Cataclysmic events, sudden and powerful, affecting or posing a real threat for many people.

2) Personal losses, physical illness, surgery, are affection, such as the loss of member of the family, a friend, etc.

3) The third group is what one commonly refers to as the "daily hassles," low-grade stressors, however an intrinsic part of life in the environment of the family, the community, or at work.

For an individual, stress encompasses all the effects following exposure to stressors. In other words, stress is additive and the result of all the experiences accumulated by the person. Therefore low term stress will be also added to the major stress of a disaster.

III. THE HUMAN EXPERIENCE OF STRESS

The stressor alone does not determine the response to stress. Indeed, each stressful stimulus is **appraised** by the person as soon as it has been sensorially grasped. This starts the first part of a two step mechanism proceeding in the brain at very high speed, therefore escaping the normal and slower paths of cognitive and truly experiential processes. During this first stage, global and rapid assessment of the resulting situation is made in view of a quick action. It proceeds unconsciously, out of awareness according to specific criteria different for each individual. These criteria have been learned and are a part of the internal resources of adaptation and protection of the person toward the environment. They can be human and cultural values, fragments of formal knowledge, past experiences of life, models, coping strategies with an outcome perceived as effective, etc.

The global appreciation of the stimulus can also be called "perception of the stimulus." It is why the list of stressors or agents provoking a stress reaction is endless since in fact the elicited response **is a response not to the true stimulus but to the perception of that stimulus by the person.**

Just as rapidly as the assessment of the stimulus(i) is made, one or several emotions are generated. Emotions and feelings are the inner force generated by each appraisal. Often, given the speed of transmission of the nervous influx, they stay out of awareness, but they will dictate the strategy of behavior and action unless, after setting aside time for reflection, another analysis of the real situation is carried out and a better coping scheme devised. Another way to change the reaction to the first perception is by training. In that case, the best immediate response to a given condition has been learned and now a part the resources of the individual. The latter learned reflex takes over the first.

As action is taken, we are evaluating ourself and our effectiveness constantly to cope with the situation according to standards deeply embedded in our personality. This mechanism generates another set of emotions which on their turn will initiate other emotions and feelings. The process is endless and every time mobilizes more of the neurone synthesized neurotransmitters and entails more work for the brain cells and the rest of the body. As these reactions proceed involuntarily, they belong to the category of reflexes.

IV. SUBSTANCES INVOLVED IN THE STRESS REACTION

It is not the purpose of this chapter to dwell longer on the substances involved in the triggering of the stress response. A few have been identified but the intricate pathways of their actions is far from being known. However, it is safe to suggest that the psychological onset of the stress reaction and the stress reaction itself involve several mediators, among them powerful neurotransmitters synthesized by the cells of specific areas of the brain and hormones. Their action involves the entire body.

Experiences carried out on monkeys show that a rapid rise of the ambient temperature provokes a strong increase of the epinephrin level in their blood. Conversely, a slow rise of the temperature, unnoticed by the animal does not provoke any change.

In the human being, for example, a moderate physical exercise results in an increase of plasma norepinephrine twice as high as that of epinephrin, whereas public speaking, which requires no real physical exercise, boosts the level of plasma epinephrine three times as high as the one measured during exercise.

Of course, these results are not even reflecting the complexity of what actually takes place in the brain in terms of release of substances, correct release rates and concentration ratios between themselves, aptitude of the neurones to regenerate them, stock them, sensitivity and reactivity of the receptor sites, and other parameters that are still ignored. How can these experiments be interpreted in term of the perception of stressors and the stress reaction?

The experiments, described above, suggest that as soon as an external stimulus is recognized by the brain as novel, threatening or requiring an intervention, there is an automatic response of the organism: in the brain, substances known as neuro-transmitters are released from specific neurones in various amounts. This is a reflex, quasi instantaneous. Although no specific role can be ascribed, and we do not know which areas of the brain or which neuronal cells are involved, the following results are achieved in a matter of seconds: (6,7)

1) Release by the brain cells of effectors (amines and others) active on the autonomic nervous systems and other still unknown target organs.

2) Mobilization of the autonomic nervous system in order to prepare key physiological systems: cardio-vascular, hormonal, immunological systems, etc., for further action.

3) Some of the organs, center of these functions give us sensations that we can recognize when we become aware of them. At first, we perceive anxiety and when more time has elapsed and we are more able to sort them out, we can even describe them in terms of feelings. For instance, the pang of anxiety and threat can be experienced as a tightening, the formation of a "knot" in the stomach, an acceleration of the cardiac rhythm. If fear goes further, the muscular system gets involved and anarchic movements and shaking takes place.

4) Stimulation of cortical activity (problem solving, decision making) in view of establishing a coherent and effective plan of action for the given situation.

5) Real action on the situation and use of the resources and energies mobilized.

Every time a stimulus is perceived as important or of consequence for the person who observes it, the process described above takes place. The intensity of the reaction is not determined by the reality but **the subject's perception of the reality, that is, a distorted reality.**

The global stress response is a part of our survival instincts, a part of our inborn, natural tendencies to protect our life. It is more proper to call the action generated by the perception of the stimulus and the emotional impulse which ensues, "reaction." This would distinguish it clearly from the word "action" an act executed upon a deliberate decision of the person after reflection, examination of alternate solutions, and finally choice of the best strategy.

The emotions continuously generated in the course of the action further the excitation of the nervous cells and provide the release of more neuro-transmitters, hormones, etc. ensuring the continuity of the coping action as long as it will be necessary.

However, if the coping action(s) are sustained for too long, a period takes place during which it is more and more difficult for the organism to provide the necessary elements. Fatigue takes place as a protective mechanism and if there is still no interruption of the pattern, there is finally exhaustion, at first reversible then irreversible. To return to the case of the Marathon runner: In a normal case, after a while, feeling tired he would have very likely stopped, taken some rest and later resumed his course. However, his determination to transmit an important message, his commitment to his duty (a strongly embedded value), pushed him to ignore the message of his body and to stretch out beyond his personal limits in order to achieve what he wanted.

Stress handled correctly and in reasonable amount is good for us and stretches our limits to acquire more knowledge, more personal resources. A stress, carried beyond our limits, whatever they are; physical, cognitive or emotional, even if not always as disastrous and dramatic as that of the Marathon runner, carries almost inescapable and sometimes devastating consequences.

V. ANXIETY

If action does not follow the emotional impulse almost without delay, the release of the neuro-transmitters--this is in particular the case in the presence of a new and complex situation which requires some delay for thinking and organization--a feeling of restlessness, tightness and discomfort is experienced, pending action: this is anxiety.

VI. DISASTERS. DEFINITION AND IMPACT

There is little consensus in the literature on the basic concepts of disaster itself (8). It has been said "...a disaster is perhaps easier to recognize than it is to define."(9) Tentatively, one can describe a disaster as a sudden, unexpected and generally violent disruption of an otherwise fairly predictable environment. It has a striking physical aspect, is usually of short duration, leaves a great number of casualties (death or injuries and/or destruction). In all cases, it is beyond the normal limits of human experience. It is for everyone a tremendous loss and has long and tragic consequences.

One can further divide disasters into two categories:

1) the natural events: earthquakes, tornadoes, volcanic eruptions, flooding, etc.

2) or the disasters due to human error or technology defects: train derailment, plane crash, massive liberation of toxic gas, rupture of dams, radioactive release, collapse of an architectural structure.

Although in both cases the end results are the same: casualties and destruction, and the efforts of relief always harrowing. The perception of the disaster is different in terms of the mental and emotional consequences both for victims and rescuers.

VII. EMOTIONAL RESPONSES OF THE RESCUERS TO A DISASTER

One can identify four major emotional responses in the unfolding of the rescuers intervention:

1) Breaking of the news or the Alarm Reaction

A disaster is always sudden and unpredictable. Surprise is the first emotion associated with its occurrence. This is very important to point out because although rescuers have prepared their skills for intervention, at the time of the intervention, unconsciously an enormous mobilization of nervous energy takes place prompted by the sense of emergency of the relief to be given, and the fact that disaster strikes and takes everyone aback. No matter how well prepared, there is always confusion and disorientation lurking since information is always scarce, adding the extra stress of anticipated difficulties and waste of time in a situation where often waste of time means loss of human lives. There is a lot of nervous energy built up and dissipated in damaging anxiety due to the lack of information.

2) **Mobilization and organization phase: on the way to the disaster site**

Depending upon the amplitude of the disaster, the conditions to reach the site will be more or less easy. It is obvious that the slower and the more laborious the arrival on site, the more emotionally taxing.

Right at this stage, there is an important offshoot of the disaster exercises. If the teams are well trained, the rescue plan well established and exercises have been previously carried out, the coordination is well organized, the emotional relief for the workers will be significant. They will be confident that their assistance will be as efficient as possible. Trained workers having already participated in relief efforts as a result, are calm and collected. This concentration before the effort helps the conservation of energy by opposition to the case of non-seasoned rescuers for whom a disaster is still a novelty or who did not take part in exercises.

3) **The actual confrontation or Action phase**

Many reports of disaster mention a feeling of shock by observers at the sight of the disaster area and a particular perception of the sounds. Silence, human screams, etc. Every sensorial stimulus is seared in the memory of the rescuers and expressed in terms reflecting the close association with shock and death. At this stage, although prey to a lot of emotions, the worker quickly and actively engages in the rescue tasks.

Beside the work itself, which most of the time is hard and difficult, the circumstances of the relief can be particularly demanding and strenuous.

- daylight or obscurity of night, extremes in temperature, weather, conditions, mud, water, etc...
- frustrations generated by the lack of coordination, lack or ambiguity of information, of communication and the irritability of fellow rescuers generated by fatigue.
- circumstances, such as the difficulties of decisions too hastily made on site (amputation of limbs in order to get the victim out of debris, the choice in the order of saving victims, etc.) All these circumstances are particularly exacting and take an enormous toll on the rescuers physically and emotionally.

Table I on the following page shows the conditions in which a few disasters took place.

TABLE I.

CAUSES OF DISASTER	CONDITIONS OF RESCUE	HUMAN/CASUALTIES
Breaking of a dam. Human negligence. No maintenance.	Muddy water used in coal processing.	Heavy
Human negligence during maintenance.	Extreme heat. Sight of charred and mutilated bodies.	Heavy
Flaw in design and building.	Heat and thunderstorm. Obscurity. Water due to damaged water pipes. Rescue by excavation.	Heavy
Human negligence. Insufficient de-icing of plane.	Extreme cold. Rescue in the partially frozen Potomac river.	Numerous
Human negligence.	Fear of an accident getting out of control with high potential danger. Evacuation.	None
Natural disaster.	Education and evacuation.	Light
Human negligence in preparing an experiment.	Dangerous technology out of control. Deadly risks impossible to detect.	High
Natural disaster with human negligence: faulty engineering.	High risks for rescuers. Excavation in concrete with danger of collapsing structures.	Numerous

SITE OF DISASTER	YEAR	NATURE OF DISASTER
Buffalo Creek West Virginia	1976	Breaking of a dam.
United Airline DC 10 Crash Chicago O'Hare	1979	Crash on takeoff.
Hyatt Hotel Kansas City	1981 (Summer)	Collapse of a Skywalk 1500 persons attending a tea dance.
Air Florida Flight 90 Washington DC	1982 (Winter)	Crash during takeoff.
Three Mile Island	1979	Interruption of the cooling system of a nuclear reactor.

SITE OF DISASTER	YEAR	NATURE OF DISASTER
Mount St. Helen	1980	Volcanic eruption.
Chernobyl	1982	Melting down of nuclear reactors.
San Francisco	1989	Earthquake. Collapse of double-deck highway.

TABLE II

1. <u>Alarm Reaction</u>.

   Surprise
   Anxiety
   Disorientation and confusion.
   Sense of emergency.

2. <u>Going to the disaster site</u>.

   Bracing of self.
   Anticipation.
   Impatience.
   Anxiety.
   Sense of emergency.

3. <u>Confrontation</u>.

   Surprise and shock at sight, noises or silence.
   Excitement.
   Overwhelming and confused emotions
   Awareness of personal danger
   Anger
   Hatred
   Guilt
   Grief
   Disgust
   Despair
   Denial

4. <u>Aftermath of disaster</u>.

   Fatigue
   Profound emotional stirring (aware or unaware)
   Confusion
   Regrets
   Denial
   Grief
   Anger
   Guilt
   Despair
   Burden of coping with other areas of personal life.

Furthermore, there is always a sense of the personal danger involved: the more hazardous, the more unpredictable and mysterious the situation, the harder emotionally. There has been no extensive writing on Chernobyl and the melting down of the nuclear reactors, but from the upheaval a minor accident like Three Mile Island has generated, it is easy to extrapolate what must have been the level of anxiety of the relief workers. They knew the danger of radioactivity but were ignorant of the extent of their exposure to the radiations and very rightly were expecting to develop in the future a disease associated with radioactivity.

The length of time involved is another critical factor. One can predict that the longer the time at work or the more overtime, the more likely an individual will undergo a burn-out.

Finally, whether the disaster is a natural calamity or a man-made disaster is of importance. Indeed, although the magnitude of natural disasters such as earthquake, tornadoes, flooding, or volcanic eruptions can be awesome; there is a general sense of acceptation of the event as something rare, as an unavoidable calamity linked to our fate on planet Earth. Research and technology try to make these events more predictable and to minimize their effects by information and evacuation. (13)

This is not so with man-made disasters. One believes that when man builds something, he is in control of the functioning and the consequences of the changes he introduces in the environment. Cases of the contrary are unfortunately numerous: no maintenance program (case of the Buffalo Creek Dam), or not properly conducted (Air Crash of United Airlines DC 10 in Chicago O'Hare Airport), construction flaws, (the collapse of the highway during the 1989 earthquake in San Francisco). The list is long. In some of these disasters, there are warnings, usually ignored until the dramatic happening takes place.

The normal emotional reaction which ensues is anger, a monstrous anger; in certain cases--rage against the devastation and the loss of human lives. Frequently associated with anger is another profound emotion: helplessness.

I want to insist particularly on the latter since in fact, it looms large on the whole field of catastrophes. A disaster is beyond the normal scale of human intervention and there is indeed a normal feeling of it being beyond human power. Experiencing helplessness can be a very intense and particularly devastating reaction, especially if in the past of the person it reactivates traumatic experiences. It can have a strong bearing in the development of the post-traumatic stress syndrome. Helplessness also exacerbates the power of the other emotions. For instance, helplessness and anger becomes rage and desire for revenge, sadness, despair, etc...leading toward an even more active release of neurotransmitters and favoring nervous exhaustion.

Another powerful emotion felt by almost all workers is guilt: guilt not to have worked a little extra, guilt not to have rescued one victim faster than another, guilt to be alive when children or others are dead, etc. The reasons are endless. Guilt as an obsessive feeling stems from an unaware often denied anger against the multiple circumstances of a disaster (10). Table II summarizes the emotions and feelings elicited during the confrontation stage.

TABLE III

Long term psychological, physical and behavioral consequences for the individual engaged in a relief effort after a disaster.

A) **Emotional problems.**

Anxiety and depression.

Frequent and uncontrollable experiences of feelings of anger, guilt and fear.

Reliving or flashbacks scenes of the catastrophic events.

Irritability and emotional outbursts leading to conflicts in the family or within the social circles of like or at work. The consequences of these behaviors on turn is to increase the stress of the person.

Sleep disturbances and nightmares.

Decrease of sexual appetite.

B) **Inappropriate behaviors stemming from emotional difficulties related to the trauma.**

Alcoholism.

Addiction to "sleeping pills."

Fatigue, dizziness, apathy, burn-out syndrome.

Aggressive behavior.

Excessive verbal expression: need to talk over and over about the event, sharp criticisms of the hierachy, particularly in the case of man-made disasters, excessive complaints, etc.

Development of obsessive or compulsive avoidance, or even phobic behavior.

C) **Psychosomatic syndromes.**

One can find in this category any of the classical psychosomatic syndromes, in particular; irritation of the gastro-intestinal tract, lower back pain, headaches (without organic findings), etc.

Complications of pre-existing medical problems can also take place.

D) **Disturbances of the cognitive functions.**

Distractibility.

Decrease of ability to think clearly and master a task.

Decrease of job efficiency and sense of responsibility.

Frequent sense of doubt about self-worth, capability and responsibility.

4) Aftermath of the disaster or let-down phase

It would be very wrong to think that because rescue workers are trained to bring relief, they do not suffer any aftermath in terms of mental distress. Even if they are not linked in any way to the victims, as we have seen, their emotional reactions are genuine. They have been for a long time discounted and ignored on the basis that: "These people are professional, they are used to it." In fact, no one "gets used to a disaster," given the fact that for a normal person, death and suffering can be encountered and accepted only within certain limits. There is a big difference between rescuing a widely distributed number of dead and injured people from car accidents for a whole year, and what would be the impact of the same number of people dead or injured altogether at the same time and at the same place.

The experience of mass casualties and injuries is one which the human being is not and never will be ready to acquiesce to easily. To see the loss of life in the others is a reminder of our own death. As it has been often said "No one who sees a disaster is untouched by it." Aren't mass casualties provoked by war or extermination camps referred as monstrous, not human?

Talking about the DC 10 crash of Chicago, J. Duffy (11) made this comment about the rescuers: "To suggest that these individuals are trained to walk among the carnage, burning human tissue, skulls, body parts, is ludicrous." No matter how trained and efficient they are, the workers of the relief teams endure events beyond normal emotional tolerance, along with conditions physically very strenuous.

It is therefore not astonishing that, eight weeks after the crash of Air Florida Flight 90 in Washington DC, rescuers were still experiencing a great number of the symptoms describes in Table III. This list, far from exhaustive, shows the various consequences of acute and excessive stress. These problems are not limited to the rescuer himself but provoke serious difficulties in his family, at work and in the social interactions.

TAKING CARE OF THE EMERGENCY TEAMS AFTER A DISASTER

Who needs help? For the reasons mentioned above: everyone. There has been and there is still a profound resistance in some groups to "healing the helpers."(12) Indeed some of the rescuers are usually perceived as strong persons and it is a part of their subculture to see themselves as such. By asking for emotional support, they fear that their image and that of rescuers could be shattered. This is even more true if there has been criticisms by some of the victims or the media, such as, "slow to respond" or "lacking of coordination." Denial, entrenchment behind a wall of silence, behind alcohol, or sinking into depression seem to them more acceptable outcomes. There is unfortunately only a slow departure from these attitudes.

Although severe emotional impairment is not often encountered as a consequence of participation in relief efforts, a survey (12) of a group of 360 emergency workers of all types: fire fighters, paramedics, emergency medical technicians, police officers, nurses in emergency room or intensive care units, admitted that 86.9% of them had been physically and emotionally affected by their work; among them, 22% felt burnt out. Moreover, 93.3% consider that debriefing sessions (13) at the end of each day of work during a disaster were necessary, helping the venting of anxiety. During the post-disaster period, support groups brought them relief and they consider them as essential since they alleviate the burden left on the family alone to cope with the symptoms depicted in Table III.

WHO IS A GOOD CANDIDATE FOR MEMBERSHIP IN A RESCUE TEAM?

This is a question which, if answered, would solve many problems. It is without doubt that some workers are coping with their tasks in a better fashion than others, and that some individuals seem to have a natural protection which leads them to be less affected by traumatic experiences than some others. The difference resides in the personal resources of the individual. However, personality factors favoring a better handling of disaster situation are still unknown.

So far, too little research has been made in this complex area. However, in the studies done on victims of PTSD, it seems that individuals lacking a good family support or those who went through a difficult childhood are more fragile.

Persons who want to give up this type of work or feel unfit should be encouraged to leave, thereby decreasing their own risks of mental strain. If the turn-over is "bad" for the team, at least the individuals who are staying are more "up to the work."

PREVENTIVE HELP FOR THE WORKERS

a) Creating a more responsive and supportive environment.

The rescue workers are obviously in need of special programs. In a threatened region, it would be wrong to restrict preventive assistance to the relief workers alone. Close associations should be established between the rescues teams, the health practitioners and the mental health teams. This could take place in each community during the course of an exercise for example or during informal encounters.

Too many barriers still exist between rescue personnel and mental health professionals and the population in areas of potential disasters. An excellent demonstration has been recorded in the case of the Mount St. Helens volcano eruption (14) where a program of information about the danger, first emergency help and coping by formation of self-help groups and debriefing sessions were extended to the whole population. It relieved the pressure on the emergency teams who were then able to concentrate on matters which cannot be handled by anyone else.

b) It is beyond the scope of this chapter to give the specifics of training for the emergency professionals and the part-time volunteers participating in cases of major accidents. However, the following areas should be addressed:

1. Physical training in exercise and relaxation. Awareness and explanation of extreme stress consequences which the workers can experience.

2. Stress reduction programs, especially with awareness of the physical consequences of unresolved conflicts. Awareness of one's own specific drives under stress. Making a personal plan for health and stress reduction.

3. Training in decision-making and problem-solving under stress.

4. Formation of groups used to work with a mental health professional. The latter should be **trained in the field of disaster stress** and could be the leader of the debriefing sessions held after each work day during the emergency period (13-15).

5. Participation in special workshops on assertiveness, communications skills, etc (16).

6. Encouragement to set up informal support groups.

7. Encouragement to form a spouse and family support network.

A LAST WORD

It is essential for the authorities organizing the planning of disasters to be vigilant of the problems and ways of providing communication and information to the victims' spouses; to be specific in the use of their words and to remember that a disaster because of its nature generates anxiety, confusion and disarray. The only way to alleviate these predicaments is by education, training and disaster exercises involving the participation of all. This is also the only way to ensure the best preparedness for disasters.(17)

REFERENCES

1. Diagnostic and Statistical Manual of Mental Disorders 3rd. Ed. American Psychiatric Association. Washington, DC.

2. Parad H., Resnik, H.L.P., Parad L. eds. Emergency and Disaster Management. A Mental Health Source Book. Bowie MD: Charles Press, 1976.

3. Tierney K., Baisden B., Crisis Intervention Programs for Disasters Victims in Smaller Communities. National Institute of Mental Health. Washington, D.C.: U.S. Government Printing Office, 1979.

4. Cannon W.B., Bodily Changes in Pain, Hunger, Fear and Rage. Appleton Century - Crofts Publishers. New York, 1929.

5. Selye H., The Stress of Life, McGraw Hill Publisher, New York, 1976.

6. Lazarus R.S., and Cohen J.B., Environmental Stress in Altman, I. and Wohlwill, J.F. eds. Human Behavior and Environment: Current Theory and Research, Vol.2. New York Plenum, 1977, p. 89-127.

7. Lazarus R.S., Psychological Stress and the Coping Process. McGraw Hill, New York, 1966.

8. Quarantelli E.L., in Disasters and Mental Health: Selected Contemporary Perspectives, 1985. National Institute of Mental Health, B.J. Sowder ed.

9. Barkun M., Disaster and the Millenium, New Haven, Conn.: Yale University Press, 1974.

10. Perls F., Hefferline R.F., Goodman P., Gestalt Therapy, Dell Publishing Company, Inc. New York, 1951.

11. Quote from J.C. Duffy in The Washington Post July 9, 1979, in "Air Crash Rescue Workers Are Also Victims" by B.D. Colen.

12. Mitchell J.T. Role Stressors and Support for Emergency Workers. Proceedings from a 1984 workshop. Center for Mental Health Studies of Emergencies. National Institute of Mental Health. 1985. Rockville (MD) U.S.A.

13. Mitchell J.T. Journal of Emergency Medical Services 8, 36-39, (1983).

14. Shore J.H., Tatum E.L., Vollmer W.M., Am.J.Pub. Health 76, Supp. (1986), 76-83.

15. Farberow N., Training Manual for Human Service Workers in Major Disasters. National Institute of Health. Washington, DC: U.S. Government Printing Office, 1983.

16. Disaster Work and Mental Health: Prevention and Control of Stress Among Workers. Center for Mental Health Studies of Emergencies. National Institute of Mental Health. Rockville (MD). 1985.

17. Innovations in Mental Health Services to Disaster Victims. Center for Mental Health Studies of Emergencies, Lystad M., ed. National Institute of Mental Health. Rockville (MD) U.S.A.

ROLE AND FUNCTION OF ANTIPOISON CENTERS IN TOXICOLOGICAL EMERGENCY AND DISASTER

S.I. Magalini, M.D.
A. Barelli, M.D.

Clinical Toxicology Department
University Cattolica del Sacro Cuore - Rome, Italy

Toxicological disasters, over the last few decades, are unfortunately becoming increasingly more frequent.

In June 1974 an explosion occurred in the Nypro plant at Flixborough, United Kingdom. Twenty-nine people were killed and over 100 injured.

In December 1984 45 metric tons of methyl isocianate escaped from a pesticide warehouse in Bhopal, India. The toxic gas spread quickly over the adjacent residential area, killing many people instantly and poisoning a large number of others. An estimated 2500 died, and up to 100,000 were poisoned.

In November 1984, a liquified gas explosion in Mexico City caused 450 deaths and 4250 others were seriously injured.

It is disasters like these, and the many others that have occurred all over the world, that have made social and medical authorities particularly concerned about chemical accidents. The consequences of some toxicological disasters for a community can be disastrous for many years to come.

A large number of problems arise with the task of assisting the victims of toxicological disasters. The "therapeutical" measures that must be applied as soon as possible after the accident has occurred greatly stress social and medical services and test the capabilities of those structures involved in managing the event.

Taking into account the preventive activities that presumably had been carried out before the occurrence of the accident, there are four kinds of services involved in toxicological disaster management:

- services for prevention;
- services for information;
- services with primarily diagnostic and therapeutical aims;
- services with organization and coordination purposes. Naturally this is a flexible subdivision, since most events will involve more than one service.

Health and Medical Aspects of Disaster Preparedness
Edited by J.C. Duffy
Plenum Press, New York, 1990

According to us Antipoison Centers must be involved in all sectors of routine and disaster emergency plans, because of the enormous number of toxic substances and of the numerous mechanisms of action through which they may exert their activity.

As far as prevention is concerned, continuously updated maps of the sites where toxic substances are produced, stored or employed, must be drawn. Furthermore, it is necessary to collect and make available specific documentation on the nature of toxic substances used in large quantities, and on the metabolities formed during their production, those derived from accidental events, or after their use, as is happening with products currently employed in agriculture.

Periodic or better still, continuous monitoring of air, water, and soil for the presence of poisons, is another fundamental and efficient aspect of prevention.

All information should then be integrated to draw a sort of "territorial toxic map"; the role of local communities and authorities is very important for its constant updating.

Apart from the "territorial mapping," local communities will need another sort of information: the so called "hazard mapping." Studies of previous toxicological disasters will ensure preplanning based on experience, including the use of methods developed in epidemiology and statistics. For this purpose data bases, community profiles, assessment of need for protocols and evaluation methodology should be made available.

In managing a toxicological disaster, the main goal of the information services is to provide in real time detailed reports concerning the probable nature of the poison, the quantity and quality of its (their) metabolities and relative first aid measures. We have met with several difficulties in building up a large and efficient toxic data bank which would provide in real time this type of information at the site of accident of poisoning both in routine emergency and in disaster situations. They have been:

- the large number of data required to identify a poison;

- the synonyms of basic products and commercial preparations; and

- the need for continuous data bank updating with new products and new knowledge accumulating daily.

All these difficulties dictated the utilization of computerized systems that, employing special programs for data storage and elaboration, makes it possible to perform an immediate differential toxicological diagnosis and to indicate in real time specific therapeutical intervention.

From a technical point of view the realization of a computerized information system needs:

a) a data bank design

b) the establishment of systems for updating modalities

c) the relative software and hardware (data collection and management)

d) the training of personnel, medical and non, for data input and retrieval.

To solve these problems, various programs have been developed and tested around the world. It was decided in our group that the only feasible answer (since 1973) was the creation of a data bank on mechanographic basis and direct access through terminals.

Although the initial activity of our Antipoison Center commenced in 1970, the real onset of the direct utilization of the electronic system began in 1973, after three years of study and programming.

From then on, the hardware and software have been constantly updated to better respond to the targets indicated. Our computerized system, employing data elaboration, thus making it possible to perform an immediate differential diagnosis and to indicate in "real time" specific therapeutic interventions.

The computer is able to scan voluminous files of data at quite a high speed. Furthermore, it offers the means to generate and maintain these files or "data bases" and to archive them on direct-access devices. Data base handling and information retrieval can be performed on line, using terminals or by batch processing. We usually obtain our answer by keyboard manual input.

The possibilities offered by this computerized system are multiple and the search may be initiated starting from one of the following inputs:

- number
- product category
- brand name
- chemical name
- use
- manufacturer
- toxicity
- chronic toxicity
- symptoms
- treatment
- references

In Fig. 1 is shown an example of a toxicological card concerning propylacetate.

The search may be carried out by using one of these data or several at the same time, so limiting the range of research and shortening the time required to obtain the specific information needed.

The information is extremely useful for making a diagnosis and on giving advice as to the eventual treatment to be followed.

CODE	200094
PRODUCT TYPE	Industrial solvent
USE	Solvent
PRODUCT NAME	Propylacetate
PHYSICAL CHARACTERISTICS	Liquid, odor of pears, low solubility in water Solvent for resin, cellulose derivates, plastics
TOXICITY	Estimated lethal dose in Humans 50g MAC 200 ppm Toxic form inhalation and ingestion; may be irritating to skin and mucous membranes and high narcotic
SYMPTOMS	Ingestion: nausea, vomiting, pyrosis Inhalation: narcotic effect
CHRONIC TOXICITY	Experimental: irritation of tracheal and bronchial mucous membranes. Fatty liver.
THERAPY	Ingestion: gastric lavage: antacids Inhalation: respiratory assistance Skin or eyes contact: wash with running water
REFERENCES	2,3,8,29,36

Fig. 1

Access to the data bank at the present time is possible for about 9,000 product names, 6,500 generic or chemical names, 630 plants and animals and their common or scientific denominations, 268 different uses, 400 symptoms, either directly by one of the above inputs or indirectly by different combinations of them.

A second data bank (clinical cases) is dedicated to the storage of clinical information relative to all cases assisted by the center.

In the clinical archive the following data are stored:

- date
- number
- patient demographic data
- country
- modality of poisoning;
- date and period of admission
- chemio-merceological data on the poison responsible
- quantity of toxic agent
- symptoms
- diagnostic procedures carried out
- treatment carried out
- hospitalization time outcome

The structuring of the center with this double archive allows access to the "basic data archive" so facilitating diagnosis and the identification of specific treatment, and at the same time the storage of data on each clinical case assisted: the continuous confrontation of the two archives results in the permanent updating of the "basic data archive." In this way the latter does not represent a static source of information (collected from literature, manufactures information, etc.) but a dynamic unity continuously modified by actual clinical events that confirm or continuously modify the quality of the basic data.

The elaboration of the clinical data provides, in addition, accurate, detailed, statistical epidemiological analysis in function of various parameters, for instance:

- geographic area distribution of incidents;
- frequency of different types of poisoning;
- demographic data/frequency/type of poisoning.

These data allow the identification of specific risks and the planning and adoption of generic and specific preventive measures.

From the time of its opening, the center has answered to a progressively increasing number of calls, from the town area and from the national territory, coming from laymen, physicians and health facilities, and has provided diagnostic identification of poisons and subsequent therapeutic measures even in instances of massive poisoning.

The service is operative 24 hours a day. During the past few years, APCs have been set up in Genova, Bologna, Chieti, Napoli and Catania connected through terminals with our data banks.

These peripheral or satellite units present a double characteristic: the access to a large amount of immediate information already stored and the collection of clinical data for selected geographic areas.

Each connected Center has full autonomy in final clinical decisions and can generate independent banks of their own cases, needed for identifications and eventual statistic-epidemiological studies of their particular area epidemiology.

In the initial phase, the APC plans and develops the diagnostic and therapeutical objectives and procedures for each single toxic agent or various combinations in toxicological disaster management.

The treatment of critical patients, in life-threatening situations, is benefiting from all the fast developing methods and techniques of Intensive Care, such as the monitoring of vital and metabolic functions, computerized management of the enormous bulk of data on the nature of injuries, on diagnostic procedures and on specific therapeutic interventions.

A primary role of the APC concerning this aspect is planning and coordinating specific diagnostic and therapeutical procedures that the critical poisoned patient needs.

For this purpose the clinical archive is available in real time and provides all the information concerning both the adequate therapeutical measures and unusual clinical pictures.

Furthermore laboratory tests often assume a primary role.

In our laboratory the data bank is interfaced with analytic instrumentation and the computerized system allows the ready chemical analytic identification of poisons with diagrams of flux, initiated by an already known or then identified basic physio-chemical characteristic of the suspected poison.

Since the number of potentially toxic agents, and all relative information is so vast, it is impossible to carry out a screening without an organized pattern that follows logically arranged steps (flow chart or algorithm).

The poison may be known, unknown or simply suspect.

In these three situations the diagnostic challenges is essentially different. For instance in the first case, knowing the agent and utilizing the anamnestic data, the symptoms and the clinical pathological data, specific treatment may be immediately identified through the supporting system of the already mentioned "information data bank."

The successive specific toxicological analyses will be directed merely to confirm and/or to evaluate the amount of toxic agent in the body and its time of clearance, for planning and carrying out further specific treatment.

Finally we want to deal with the organization and coordination problems involving the APC.

Unfortunately in our country, Emergency Departments aren't working at their potential best. Consequently the organization and coordinative task of the APC is currently overloaded by the inefficiency of most Emergency Departments. Our aim is to increase the availability of such medical services and further improve the coordination between the APC and the other branches of the E.M.S., both at a national level, as we already have done in our country, and at an international level, for instance among the NATO countries.

INJURY PATTERNS ASSOCIATED WITH EARTHQUAKES

Douglas A. Rund, M.D.
Gregg S. Pollander

Ohio State University
Columbus, Ohio

INTRODUCTION

Major earthquakes create disaster conditions because the resulting structural collapse causes significant morbidity and mortality. An estimated 15 million deaths have been caused by earthquakes since the beginning of recorded history.(1) Earthquakes have caused an average of 11,250 deaths per year for the last 40 years(2) accounting for 37% of all deaths caused by disaster.(3) In addition to the injury and death caused at the time of the earth movement itself, an earthquake disrupts the community's capacity to respond effectively. Transportation, communications, and health care systems are typically damaged significantly in the hours and days following the event. As a result, national and international assistance is usually required, since the salvage rate for victims unrescued from a collapsed structure decreases steadily after the first 24 hours after entrapment, international assistance teams and equipment should be on site within one or two days. Unfortunately this kind of response time is rarely possible under present conditions.

We propose that pre-planning for response to specific types of disaster will reduce response time for provision of national and international aid. Knowledge of specific injuries usually associated with a given form of disaster makes possible the selection of hospital teams and assembly of equipment well in advance of a disaster. One can, for instance, then calculate the need (quantities and amounts) for orthopedic and neurosurgical equipment, the number of operating room hours required, number of surgeons and nurses necessary to accomplish required procedures, etc.

We attempted to discover such information by reviewing published reports of six major earthquakes occurring over the past 30 years. The data reported here show that, although some crude generalization can be made about types of injury, the lack of a uniform data collection strategy makes comparisons difficult.

In 1963, Saidi attempted to classify and quantitate injuries resulting from the 1962 earthquake in Iran(4) under the category, "other causes." The "crush syndrome" often thought to be a major concern following earthquake was not listed as a major feature of injury in this report. He was unable to report on all injuries because of the absence of accurate data. As an illustration, however, he reported one hospital's experience from the 1960 earthquake shown in Table 1. One notes a rather large number of fractures as well as medical problems that include dehydration and gastroenteritis.

De Ville de Goyet, et.al., reported injuries from an earthquake in Guatemala.(5) Occurring on February 4, 1976, at 3:02 a.m., the earthquake measured 7.5 on the Richter Scale. Destruction spread over a vast region including hilly terrain containing isolated villages and small cities. In some areas where adobe construction predominated, 90% of homes were totally destroyed. Eighteen days after the impact, the death toll measured 22,778 and the number of injuries was estimated at 76,504. Although the injury data reported for this earthquake were among the most complete at that time, the authors reported that "the reliability of the reporting system under emergency conditions was very low." Data included patients attending mobile clinics for chronic problems and in some areas it was only possible to make a "rough guess" as to the number of injured requiring care. Citing only three studies in the literature up until that time, the authors of the study noted that "scientific literature on various earthquake related lesions is scanty." The best estimates about type and distribution of lesions causing morbidity following the Guatemalan earthquake are one hospital's data presented in Table 2. The major weakness in this effort to classify and report injuries is the fact that greater than 75% of the injuries were not specified as to type.

Ortiz, et.al.,(6) published more comprehensive injury data in 1986. The authors studied injury types and distribution of injury following the 3 March 1985 earthquake in Chile measuring 7.8 on Richter Scale. A total of 1,623 injuries were reported and distributed among men and women as shown in Table 3. Though the authors admit "the information contained in this work constitutes neither a universal nor a representative sample of the injured," it represents a more sophisticated attempt to report morbidity and mortality following earthquakes.

In 1983 Gueri, et.al., published data about injuries sustained in the 1979 earthquake in Tumaco, Colombia, which measured 7.9 on the Richter scale.(7) In addition to hospital data, the authors drew a sample of 560 households from a population of 200,000 persons. An interview of a responsible member of the household was conducted by a member of the health service interview team. The subject of the interview concerned injuries and deaths associated with the earthquake. In this somewhat less chaotic situation, it was hoped that a more complete picture of injury type, magnitude and extent could be determined. The injuries reported by distribution to body part are shown in Table 4. This study also went on to report distribution of cause of death, death by age group, and location of person at time of injury.

De Bruycker, et al, surveyed households in selected Italian villages after the 1980 earthquake.(8) The authors listed the major injuries in patients with multiple injuries. As in the Gueri study, the populationbased sampling technique improved the accuracy of data collected. With regard to type of injury, the authors reported the following percentages: lacerations 42, contusions 26, fractures 18.9, and "cuts" 9.7. Anatomic sites of injury were the following: legs, 39%; head, 23.2%; chest, 18.9%; arms, 16.4%; and pelvis, 2.5%. The ability to walk immediately after the incident was measured as a rough index of injury severity: 44.5% could walk without assistance, 22.8% required assistance, and 32.7% could not walk. Thirty-two percent of the injured patients were transported directly to a medical facility.

Noji, et.al,. reported morbidity data for the 1988 earthquake in Soviet Armenia (Table 5).(9) Several aspects of the data deserve special mention.

The data seem to give better information regarding types of injury that previously published. One also notes a rather substantial percentage (11%) of patients with "crush syndrome," a condition causing massive trauma to muscle and bone, sometimes causing death within a few days from electrolyte inbalance and a cause of renal failure which led to the Soviet request for dialysis capability following the Armenian earthquake.

The most striking feature of the data found in the literature is its non-uniformity. This is obvious when one scans the injury categories listed in Tables 1 through 5. While there may be local factors such as population density and quality of housing construction that affect earthquake morbidity from incident to incident, the classification schemes themselves vary from author to author. The absence of an international classification and coding scheme for injuries sustained in earthquakes make it difficult to plan medical assistance packages, especially when medical needs are greatest in the first 24 hours following the after impact.(10) Injury classification data should ideally include the following information: all sites of major injury in an individual (not just the primary injury), whether or not the patient needs a specialized care facility (e.g., hospital, operating room, burn unit, etc.), and what types of medical personnel are most likely to be helpful (e.g., emergency physicians, general surgeons, orthopedic surgeons, neurosurgeons, etc.). From the proper kinds of injury data, one should be able to determine the types of supplies and equipment needed to care for the various casualties. This is possible only in the most general terms when one actually reviews the kind of data found in the literature.

The development of an international injury classification scheme and a strategy for accurate data collection would be of great benefit in the development of international disaster aid programs. Organizations already involved in international disaster assistance should be able to initiate the development of this program.

Table 1. Types of injuries in the 1960 Iranian earthquake. (From Saidi, F. "The 1962 Earthquake in Iran - Some Medical and Social Aspects." The New England Journal of Medicine, 1963, 268:929-932.)

Injury	Number of cases
Fractures of extremities (single or multiple)	49
Vertebral fractures	10
Pelvic fractures	7
Chest Injuries	10
Face and head injuries	9
Minor injuries, dehydration and gastroenteritis	26

Table 2. Leisons observed in patients admitted to the Jalapa Hospital during the day following the earthquake in Guatemala, 1976. (From De Ville de Goyet, et.al. "Earthquake in Guatemala: Epidemiologic Evaluation of the Relief Effort." <u>Pan American Health Organization Bulletin</u>, 1976, Vol. X, 95-109.)

Reason for admission	No. of patients affected	% of total patients
Fractured pelvis	4	2.5
Fractured clavicle	18	11.5
Fractured of the lower extremities	10	6.4
Fracture of the upper extremities	5	3.2
Other causes	120	76.4
Total	157	100.0

Table 3. Distribution of those injured by the earthquake of 3rd March 1985 in Columbia, by type of injury and sex. (From Ortiz, M.R., et.al. "Brief Description of the Effects on Health of the Earthquake of 3rd March 1985 - Chile." Disasters, 1986, 10:125-140.)

Type of Injury	Sex			Total	%
	Male	Female	Unknown		
Fracture of the skull and bones of the face	10	4	2	16	1.0
Fracture of the cervical and dorsal vertebrae	19	14	4	37	2.3
Fracture of the upper extremity	34	44	2	80	4.9
Fracture of the lower extremity	71	110	8	189	12.3
Dislocation	8	4	---	12	0.8
Sprains and tears	67	72	---	139	8.5
Intracraneal injury without fracture	37	56	2	95	5.7
Internal injury to chest, abdomen and pelvis	3	1	---	4	0.2
Wound of the head, neck and trunk	122	97	---	219	13.2
Wound of the upper extremity	74	47	1	122	8.2
Wound of the lower extremity	101	114	2	217	13.3
Superficial injury	3	5	---	8	0.5
Contusion without alteration of the skin	192	214	1	407	23.5
Bruises	3	4	---	7	0.4
Injury to the nerves and spinal column	6	1	---	7	0.4
Complications of unspecified injury	11	5	---	16	1.0
Others	23	19	6	48	3.8
Total	784	811	28	1,623	100.0
Percent	48.3	50.0	1.7	100	

Table 4. Injury distribution by type, Tumaco, Colombia, 1979. (From Gueri, M., et.al. "Health Implications of the Tumaco Earthquake, Colombia, 1979." Disasters, 1983, 7:174-179.)

Location	Number	Percentage
Head	20	8.9
Face	27	12.1
Trunk	33	14.8
Upper limbs	11	4.9
Lower Limbs	87	39.0
Nervous System	3	1.3
Abortion	3	1.3
Multiple	32	14.3
Spinal Column	7	3.1
Total	223	100.0

Table 5. Injury distribution by type, Soviet Armenia, 1988, as reported to Ministry of Health as 12/21/88. From Noji, E.K., et.al, Mortality and Morbidity Following the 1988 Earthquake in Soviet Armenia, presented at the Society of Academic Emergency Medicine, San Diego, 1989.

Injury	Number	Percentage
Skull, facial fractures	130	2.7
Spine, torsol fractures	388	8.0
Upper extremity fractures	265	5.5
Lower extremity fractures	584	12.1
Joint dislocations	61	1.3
Brain concussion	417	8.6
Other internal head trauma	173	3.6
Open head, facial wounds	320	6.6
Traumatic amputations, arms	197	4.1
Open wounds, legs	102	2.1
Traumatic amputations, legs	170	3.6
Vascular injuries	5	0.1
Superficial trauma	1203	24.9
Spinal cord injury	30	0.6
Heart, lung injuries	26	0.5
Abdominal, pelvic injuries	44	0.9
Elective amputation, arms	13	0.3
Elective amputation, legs	59	1.2
Crush Syndrome	533	11.0
Burns	56	1.2
Frostbite	4	0.08
Non-earthquake related injuries	52	1.1

References

1. Lechat, M.F. "An Epidemiologist's View of Earthquake." In Engineering Seismology and Earthquake Engineering, Ed. Julius Solnes. Noordhoff-Leiden, 11974, pp. 285-307.

2. Ganse R, Nelson J: Catalog of Significant Earthquakes, U.S. Department of Commerce - NOAA, Boulder, Colorado, 1981.

3. Shah, B.V. "Is the Environment Becoming More Hazardous?--A Global Survey 1947 to 1980." Disasters, 1983; 7:202-209.

4. Saidi, F. "The 1962 Earthquake in Iran - Some Medical and Social Aspects." The New England Journal of Medicine, 1963, 268:929-932.

5. De Ville de Goyet, et.al. "Earthquake in Guatemala: Epidemiologic Evaluation of the Relief Effort." Pan American Health Organization Bulletin, 1976, Vol. X, 95-109.

6. Ortiz, M.R., et.al. "Brief Description of the Effects on Health of the Earthquake of 3rd March 1985 - Chile." Disasters, 1986, 10:125-140.

7. Gueri, M., et.al. "Health Implications of the Tumaco Earthquake, Colombia, 1979." Disasters, 1983, 7:174-179.

8. De Bruycker M, Greco D, Lechat M. "The 1980 Earthquake in Southern Italy--Morbidity and Mortality." International Journal of Epidemiology, 1985, 14:113-117.

9. Noji, E.K., Kelen, G.D. and Oganesjan, A. "Mortality and Mobidity Following the 1988 Earthquake in Soviet Armenia," presented to the Society for Academic Emergency Medicine, San Diego, 1989.

10. Sheng, C.Y. "Medical Support in the Tangshen Earthquake: A Review of the Management of Mass Casualties and Certain Major Injuries." J. of Trauma Vol. 27(10), October, 1987.

A MULTIDISCIPLINARY APPROACH TO THE MEDICAL MANAGEMENT OF MAN-MADE AND NATURAL TOXIC DISASTERS

Peter J. Baxter, M.D.

University of Cambridge Clinical School
Addenbrooke's Hospital
Cambridge, England

INTRODUCTION

The medical management of major toxic releases involving the exposure of large numbers of people is often poorly handled, whether the route of exposure is by air, food or water (1). Toxic releases usually arise from industrial activity but natural sources, such as volcanoes, may pose similar problems. A common fault of the emergency response is the delay, for a variety of reasons, in the identification of the agent or agents involved and in evaluating the health risk posed (1). The task of health risk assessment needs to be urgently performed in a major toxic incident, but it requires a multidisciplinary approach that may be difficult to launch in an emergency or disaster. In this chapter I shall describe some of the uses and limitations of the major disciplines that need to be involved, beginning with a classical toxic disaster in the workplace as a starting point for the study of toxic releases in the community.

THE WORKPLACE AS A MODEL: THE EXAMPLE OF VINYL CHLORIDE

Information on the effects of human exposure to many industrial chemicals has been obtained by studying occupational groups. The exposures are usually much higher and over longer periods than would occur in an accidental release or from long-term environmental pollution. The health consequences of living near a toxic waste site or from consuming drinking water from an aquifer contaminated with trace amounts of a chemical are difficult, if not impossible, to quantify directly by epidemiological studies because the health risks, if they exist at all, may be too small to measure. Where possible, extrapolations can be made from studies of workplace exposures as well as from animal experiments, though for the majority of chemicals in commercial usage there is not information on toxicity available at all (2).

Vinyl chloride monomer, used to manufacture the widely used plastic poly vinyl chloride (PVC), was regarded as a safe chemical until laboratory animal studies in the early 1970s showed that it caused angiosarcoma of the liver (ASL). An urgent search for human cases in the PVC industry rapidly confirmed that the tumor occurred in workers also. The causal association with exposure to the chemical was irrefutable and a shocked industry, working with government and unions, moved quickly to impose strict controls (3). But what was the extent of the risk? As well as extrapolating from

Health and Medical Aspects of Disaster Preparedness
Edited by J.C. Duffy
Plenum Press, New York, 1990

toxicological studies the quickest way of making a preliminary assessment was to do retrospective epidemiological studies of the incidence of ASL in the population and in exposed workers. A study of all cases of ASL that could be identified to have occurred in the United Kingdom in 1963-73 showed that the tumor was indeed very rare and that there were no additional cases linked to vinyl chloride exposure other than the one that was already known about from a search of factory records (4,5). A national, retrospective cohort study of workers engaged in PVC manufacturing corroborated this conclusion (6). Similar studies were conducted in the United States (7) and other countries. Since then about 150 cases have been identified in vinyl chloride workers worldwide. All of the tumors have occurred years after heavy occupational exposure, and the risk to populations from the contamination of food or drink with vinyl chloride from PVC packaging, or from airborne emissions around PVC plants, is regarded as remote. Thus, through a major collaborative effort involving industry, government bodies and research groups, a full and rapid assessment of the health risk was made.

Vinyl chloride has become a classic story in the history of environmental hazards and, like other notable examples such as asbestos, has provided a strong impetus for investigators seeking to identify other chemical hazards. Unfortunately, experience has shown that the linking of cause and effect is seldom so clear-cut, even in industrial situations. Nevertheless similar methodological principles need to be applied to the field investigation of accidental toxic releases into the community, despite the greater practical difficulties these events pose.

TYPES OF ACCIDENTAL RELEASE

Acute chemical incidents involving water, food and drink are those in which there is a short latent period (days or weeks), or the outbreak is explosive and resembles an infectious disease. The epidemiological methods for identifying a causal agent are much the same as for an acute infectious disease outbreak, e.g., food poisoning. The incidents can be subdivided into those involving additives or contaminants (Table 1). An accident during the manufacture or supply of a product may result in a normally safe chemical additive used to improve the quality of the food being added accidentally in excess; or a new additive may have unexpected health consequences. Chemical contamination may occur during the transport of the food, drink or water to the consumer, or there may be deliberate adulteration or the illicit use of industrial chemicals in manufacturing.

Incidents involving heavy pollution of drinking water are usually rapidly identified because a change in water quality (smell or taste) is obvious to the supplier or consumer. More dangerous are those incidents involving food and drink, with the greatest impact occurring in those involving chronic exposure to contaminated food, when thousands of people may become exposed before the severity and cause of the problems become recognized. Airborne releases of chemicals may result in high acute mortality and morbidity in densely populated areas, (e.g., Bhopal in 1984), or pose concerns over chronic disease with long latency (e.g., Seveso 1976). A feature of toxic disasters is that they may cause few if any acute effects, but the greatest concern, as with vinyl chloride, can be over long-term health risks of exposure, especially carcinogenicity (Table 2). Moreover, some acute and chronic diseases caused by chemical exposure may be no different clinically or pathologically from diseases due to so-called natural causes. Long-term epidemiological studies may therefore be an essential feature of the risk assessment to determine the relationship between disease and exposure. Because so little is known about the acute and chronic effects of most chemicals, including dose responses in many, epidemiological investigations of exposed populations should be undertaken whenever possible, in both acute and chronic releases.

TYPES OF INVESTIGATIONS

1. Epidemiology

Why should epidemiology claim to be a fundamental importance in the medical management of a major toxic incident? Epidemiology is the basic scientific tool for the collection and evaluation of health data in population groups and so is widely applicable to the study of acute or chronic disorders. However, the number of adequately executed epidemiological studies in toxic incidents have been few, and the application of epidemiology to natural and man-made disasters is a relatively recent development. Two situations can arise. An outbreak of illness has occurred and there is a need to investigate or confirm the agent or agents responsible; alternatively a population has been exposed to a known chemical or mixture of chemicals and studies are required to determine whether there are any health implications. In both types of event the epidemiological investigation should be an integral part of the emergency response with information gathering as a vital part of evaluation of the hazard to health. The investigators must be charged with the task of giving rapid feedback and advice to clinicians and other decision-makers as the picture unfolds, with the disaster coordinating team able to respond to the media with valid information so that irrational public fears can be allayed and advice disseminated. It is therefore essential that the epidemiological team is on the scene and in continuous contact with the team leaders of the other disciplines involved so that information can be freely exchanged. At the eruption of Mount St Helens in the United States in 1980, the Federal Emergency Management Agency (FEMA) leaned heavily on the Centers for Disease Control (CDC) as the lead public health organization whose field team provided daily information on all health aspects related to the volcanic disaster.

The role of epidemiology may be illustrated by reference to this and another natural toxic disaster, namely the release of gas from Lake Nyos in Cameroon in 1986.

ERUPTION OF MOUNT ST. HELENS, May 18, 1989

This eruption resulted in a heavy ash fall over a widely populated area of Washington State and Idaho, which in some cities was as much as a 5-40cm deep. This was the first time in recent history that the United States had experienced such an event and it was initially thought to be the most serious natural disaster ever to have befallen the country. A description of the medical management of the public health hazard is given elsewhere (8). Much destruction had occurred around the volcano and devastating mud flows had traveled down the Tootle and Cowlitz Rivers into the Columbia River as far as Portland. Of most immediate concern to the population living in the area of major ash fall was whether the ash posed a hazard to human health, either as being toxic if ingested or inhaled, or capable of causing lung disease. Outdoor workers (e.g., emergency workers, farmers and loggers) were the most exposed but people were also concerned about the susceptibility of children. The Centers for Disease Control was contacted soon after the eruption for advice on these issues, but it had not had any experience in investigating health problems in volcanic eruptions. Furthermore no one at CDC knew where to turn for such advice, and indeed a literature search by the National Library of Medicine failed to find any useful references. A CDC team of medical epidemiologists was invited to undertake field investigations and arrived three days after the eruption, shortly before the FEMA set up its coordinating center.

CDC initiated a chemical analysis of the ash from the health viewpoint, though other organizations had also started testing for pH and leachable toxic elements. The ash did not have a high content of fluorine or heavy metals capable of intoxicating animals or man. However, over 90% of the particles were by count less than 10 microns in diameter and within the respirable range. A local laboratory investigating the crystalline silica content of the ash initially found a concentration of 20% whereas estimates by geologists suggested that there was no crystalline silica present at all. The great disparity between these findings needed to be rapidly resolved as the concentration of crystalline silica is a key characteristic for determining the fibrogenic potential of the ash and thus its ability to cause silicosis. The CDC's National Institute for Occupational Safety & Health (NIOSH) soon showed that the concentration was nearer 5-7%, but a dispute over the analytical methods continued which was eventually resolved in NIOSH's favor. Concerns over the potential carcinogenicity of the ash were allayed when laboratories failed to find asbestiform fibers or a high level of radioactivity.

In parallel with these investigations, epidemiological monitoring was established using a network of hospitals located in the areas of ash fall. The attendances of patients in the emergency departments and number of admissions to hospitals were obtained on a daily basis for those diagnoses of interest and the results were collated by the CDC team in Seattle. The data clearly showed a moderate increase in the number of attendances and admissions for respiratory disease during the ash fall period and in the days after. Not only were there very high levels of air-borne ash during the ash fall (outdoor visibility was near zero) but high levels continued for two weeks in the arid areas of mid-Washington and until the ash became compacted by rainfall. A meeting of senior chest physicians from all over Washington State held in the first days after the massive ash fall of May 18 was able to allay concerns that the ash could have serious acute respiratory effects on the basis of the early findings of the surveillance system. These findings had greater weight than reports from individual physicians which were dependent upon observations on small numbers of their own patients.

A case control study of the respiratory cases was undertaken in one of the affected cities which confirmed that attendances had been mostly for asthma and bronchitis and that many patients with known chronic respiratory disorders continued to have an exacerbation of chest problems for at least three months after the ash fall and during the persistence of the ash in the environment. In addition, rapid assessments of exposure to airborne ash were performed in groups of outdoor workers, the results of which were reassuring. In the post-disaster phase, animal studies showed that ash had only a moderate potential for causing pulmonary fibrosis compared to crystalline silica in that the hazard to outdoor workers and others was low. A 5-year cohort study of the respiratory hazard in loggers was begun by NIOSH; apart from a short-term reversible decline in lung function and a reversible increase in chest symptoms, both related to exposure, no serious effects were found. These and other studies summarized elsewhere (8) resulted in a complete evaluation of the health hazard. The emergency response has been hailed as a model of its kind and one which should be emulated in other major toxic incidents (9). The rapid response enabled FEMA to provide authoritative scientific and health information to the media thereby allaying public fears and providing advice about this unfamiliar hazard. But the medical epidemiologists' approach was the basic one which first raised the key health questions about the ash and the need for health surveillance.

GAS BURST FROM LAKE NYOS, CAMEROON, AUGUST 18, 1986

This natural disaster showed how the absence of appropriate investigation can make understanding of a toxic disaster virtually impossible (10). A huge gas release occurred at approximately 10 o'clock in the evening and killed about 1700 people living in a remote mountainous area north of the lake. A large number of cattle and other animals also died. This phenomenon was without precedent in the scientific record and much speculation ensued over the mechanism of the release and the type of gas or gases involved. A detailed epidemiological assessment using autopsy and toxicological findings would probably have been capable of resolving the scientific dispute that followed, or at least given insights into volcanic processes. It is now presumed that the gas was carbon dioxide and was released by a limnological mechanism rather that a volcanic eruption, the lake being capable of storing large amounts of CO_2 in its depths.

However, the first reports of the medical effects in victims suggested that they had been exposed to an acidic gas, which was one reason why some scientists initially believed that a mixture of gases had been released as part of a volcanic eruption from beneath the lake. It took a week after the event before the first foreign scientists arrived on the scene, by which time corpses had been buried without autopsies. For cultural reasons it was not possible to give survivors an interview-administered questionnaire or to rely upon the local tribesmen's accounts of their experiences. The only really useful medical evidence was that derived from the collation of the signs and symptoms of the hospitalized survivors (10). This epidemiological assessment showed that it was most likely that exposure had been to an asphyxiant rather than irritant gas and that the bullous skin lesions found on corpses and the "burns" on the skin of 20% of hospitalized survivors were also the consequences of such an exposure rather than effects of acidic gases. These findings gave support to the limnological hypothesis, though this is the first time that exposure to CO_2 has occurred on such a scale. This incident highlights the need for a medical task force to be urgently sent to such disasters and to begin investigations as soon as possible and before vital evidence is lost.

2. Clinical investigations

Victims of the acute or chronic health effects of a toxic release seeking medical aid may be the first indication that a major incident has occurred, particularly if the route of exposure is through food and drink, or water, as opposed to an airborne emission. Nevertheless, the clinical findings may be difficult to interpret unless an epidemiological investigation is carried out, particularly if the clinical manifestations are not pathognomonic of a toxic illness. Laymen often suppose that doctors are being obtuse when they cannot say from clinical investigations alone whether someone is suffering from a toxic exposure or not. The public also frequently believes that modern medicine has an armentarium of antidotes against almost any chemical, yet the number of chemicals whose acute effects can be neutralized in this way is less than a dozen.

The lack of specificity of chemical-induced illness was well illustrated in the toxic oil syndrome in Spain in 1981 which began with victims being admitted to hospitals with a diagnosis of atypical pneumonia at the rate of 600 a day at the peak of the outbreak, with about 20,000 people being affected overall (11). At first it was not unreasonably supposed that the cause was an infectious agent, but two to three weeks later when the routine tests for infectious agents were demonstrably negative, suspicion fell on a toxic cause. Clinicians began carefully questioning their patients for clues and a seemingly common factor was that they had consumed a type of rape seed oil bought as a cheap substitute for olive oil from street tradesmen. This clinical finding was confirmed in an epidemiological survey, but this was conducted after the association had been publicized by the media. A delayed clinical phase of the illness occurred in many who had recovered from the pneumonia and in contrast this was highly specific, being characterized by neuropathy, myopathy, siccal syndrome and scleroderma-like skin disease; many of the 600 or more deaths that have occurred were due to neuromuscular complications. The Toxic Oil Syndrome had not been recorded in the medical literature before and at present one can only speculate on the circumstances when it may be recognized again (11).

Organic mercury poisoning had been recorded in the industrial medicine literature some years before the condition dramatically reappeared in an environmental, rather than an industrial setting, at Minamata, Japan, in 1956 (12). Initially the outbreak of this unusual neurological disease was also believed to be an infection. Not until three years later was its resemblance to the industrial disease realized and in 1968 it was confirmed that the source of the organic mercury had been the local chemical factory's discharges into Minimata Bay. Fish had become contaminated with methyl mercury thereby poisoning the staple diet of poor fishermen and their families in the area, though eventually 50,000 people were believed to have been at risk (12). A Japanese physician, Harada, was able to undertake neurological surveys in fishermen's homes to detect undiagnosed cases, as the classical triad of this syndrome (constriction of visual fields, cerebellar signs and speech disturbances) could be readily detected on clinical examination. Numerous outbreaks of organic mercury poisoning have since been identified in several countries as a result of the ingestion of bread made from wheat seed dressed with organic mercury as a fungicide. Since the Minamata outbreak, the features of this poisoning are so well known that when there was an outbreak affecting thousands of people in Iraq in 1971 it was rapidly recognized. As a result the duration of exposure was only two weeks to two months, as opposed to the many years at Minamata; and the prognosis of the conditions in the two outbreaks was consequently quite different, with many cases in Iraq showing reversibility (13). Other characteristic syndromes arising from food-borne epidemics include porphyria cutanea tarda caused by hexachlorobenzene in Turkey in 1955-61 (14), and the motor neuropathy caused by tri-ortho-cresyl-phosphate which, unlike the former, has occurred in epidemics in many different countries around the world (15). In contrast, two major outbreaks of margarine disease due to a toxic additive were readily confused with a viral aetiology (erythema infectiossum) (16).

In 1968 dermatologists in the southern part of Japan were confronted with cases of an unusual skin condition which they were unable to explain. The frustrated sufferers eventually demanded that a particular edible oil - rice oil - be submitted for chemical analysis and it was soon shown that they had been poisoned by polychlorinated biphenyls (PCBs) which had leaked into the oil during its manufacture. The epidemic was defined by an epidemiological survey and it was shown that the disease known as Yusho, or "rice oil disease," had affected thousands and had systemic toxic manifestations, but had not been identified before (17). The skin condition was chloracne, a complaint that had previously only been recognized in workers exposed to certain chlorinated compounds. Chloracne has since been shown to be pathognomonic of exposure to chlorinated dibenzofurans (trace contaminants of PCBs) and chlorinated dibenzodioxins. The latter may arise as contaminants in the manufacture of 245-trichlorophenol: 2378-tetrachlorodibenzodioxin was responsible for the scare around the ICMESA chemical plant in Seveso in 1976 when the exothermic reaction went out of control and a toxic cloud descended on the area; 187 children developed chloracne (18). Thus the clinical sign of chloracne is specific to this type of toxic exposure though in mild forms it can be easily missed or confused with common blackheads on the face.

Thus, apart from a few specific conditions, clinical investigation may not by itself be alerting to a toxic illness and further investigations are usually necessary to interpret the significance of the presence or absence of clinical abnormalities. In particular, reliance upon clinical findings alone in an acute episode can be very misleading as to the true risk to health, and epidemiological surveys are often necessary adjuncts as shown above. Clinicians should therefore beware of providing snap judgements after the examination of a few victims and appreciate that their evidence is only one aspect of a much larger information-gathering exercise.

3. Pathology

Clinical findings on survivors need to be closely linked with pathological studies on those who have died in a disaster. Autopsy studies are essential for establishing the cause of death, yet the pathological abnormalities, like the clinical findings, may not be specific enough to assist in the early phases of an investigation of an acute epidemic. For instance, an outbreak of nine cases of acute hepatitis in Newbern, North Carolina, from July 7-28 1979, led to an urgent investigation being conducted by the CDC as six of the patients died from fulminant hepatitis. The pathological findings were massive hapatic necrosis with collapse of the reticular structure of the liver tissue and proliferation of the bile ducts. These appearances could have been due to infection by hepatitis B virus or a potent hepatotoxin, and so diagnostic confirmation had to await laboratory tests for hepatitis B infection, which were positive. In contrast, an outbreak of toxic jaundice in Epping, England, in 1968, due to the consumption of bread contaminated with methylene dianiline, was characterized by an unusual histological appearance as revealed by liver biopsy (19).

Failure to perform autopsies can lead to the loss of invaluable information. In the Lake Nyos disaster all the corpses soon were buried without examination, even though much could have been learned at autopsy from the appearances of the lungs and respiratory tract, and the histology of the skin lesions (10). The absence of acute inflammation of the upper respiratory tract would have been strong evidence that a mixture of acidic gases had not been involved and it was more likely to be an asphyxiant gas such as carbon dioxide. Autopsies conducted on those killed in the Mount St. Helens eruption in 1980 showed for the first time the key role played by ash in causing asphyxia among those caught in the pyroclastic flow (20). In practice, it is extremely difficult in the immediate aftermath of a disaster to coordinate search and rescue operations, so the retrieval of corpses is inevitably done in an uncoordinated way with little thought for the need to photograph and study the location and state of the corpses, including the conditions in the immediate environment. Pathological studies should not be confined to the mortuary but should incorporate forensic descriptions at the scene.

4. Laboratory

The role of the laboratory biochemist is a fundamental one in identifying the toxic agent or agents if there is doubt as to what has constituted the toxic release. Initial reports on the nature of the release should always be verified and it may be essential to undertake chemical testing to do this. This can be done through obtaining samples from the industrial process involved, the vehicle of exposure if it is water, food or drink (see Environmental Studies, below); and finally by biological monitoring of the blood, urine or tissues of those who have been exposed. Surveys of the exposed population to determine exposure should include obtaining biological specimens and these should also be routinely collected on those attending hospitals in the aftermath of a suspected or recognized toxic incident and on those who have died. These samples may need to be carefully stored for an indefinite period if a suitable analytical technique is unavailable. Thus, it was not until 1988 that it became possible to measure dioxin in serum samples of residents exposed in the Seveso incident in 1976 (21).

Analysis of biological samples from the exposed population may also provide important evidence on the extent of the spread of a chemical agent. In Michigan, USA, in 1973, dairy produce and meat became contaminated with polybrominated biphenuls (PBBs) as a result of an accidental substitution of a fire retardant containing PBBs with a feed additive for cattle (22). Analysis of human breast milk in a sample of the population showed that an estimated eight million of the 9.1 million Michigan residents were likely to have detectable body burns of PBB (23). In another incident involving the contamination of polychlorinated biphenyls in chicken feed, evidence of exposure became apparent when the egg consumption of a group of residents was correlated with PCB levels in breast milk (24). The extent of human contamination by DDT from a defunct DDT-manufacturing plant polluting a river in Triana, Alabama, was obtained by blood testing of the town's population (25).

Of great importance is the ability to relate any symptoms or signs to an objective measure of exposure as given by the concentrations of the putative agent in the urine, blood or other tissue of those exposed. The latter are important objective markers of exposure from which dose-response relationships can be derived, thereby providing what is often the best evidence for a causal relationship between exposure and effects on health. This approach is widely used in the study of occupational groups, measuring either the agent of interest directly or one of its metabolites. The value of immunological markers of exposure (also widely used in occupational medicine) was shown when strong evidence for a causal relationship between epidemics of asthma in the local population and unloading of soya beans in the docks of Barcelona was provided by a survey which found that 90% of those affected had IgE antibody to soya bean dust in their sera, a much high figure than in controls (26).

Clinicians need to know whether a patient has been exposed and if so by how much? Negative findings have an obvious value in reassurance. However, the desire to establish a level of exposure in an affected population or in individuals needs to be pursued cautiously as the labelling of healthy people as exposed or unexposed can have important social implications. For example, in the Yusho epidemic in 1968, the marriage prospects of some females known to have had exposure to PCBs were reported to have been blighted if the information was disclosed to prospective partners. Medical practitioners would also wish to include tests of organ dysfunction as a measure of exposure. Unfortunately routine hospital biochemical tests may lack adequate sensitivity and specificity for use after most toxic releases unless, of course, the victims are badly enough affected to result in their admission to hospital. Obviously such tests should be included in a survey when biological samples are being collected to evaluate the absorption of a chemical, but the results may be difficult to interpret in the absence of overt illness.

Another practical problem is when the investigators are presented with clinical signs and symptoms of an outbreak and then have to track down the toxic material responsible when the vehicle of exposure is unknown. In these circumstances the number of theoretical causal agents may be legion and schemes for the whittling down of the number of test options have been suggested (27).

6. Environmental

Environmental investigations should start at the source of a toxic release; e.g., inside the chemical plant or at the site of a fire, explosion or eruption. Access to a chemical plant if one is involved is essential at the earliest possible opportunity so that samples of reacted products can be obtained by chemical engineers, and the process studied to determine the cause of the accident. Arguments still continue whether hydrogen cyanide was involved in the release of methyl isocyanate from the Union Carbide Plant at Bhopal and this could possibly have been resolved if more extensive testing had been performed soon after the release. As it was, no hydrogen cyanide residue was detected in any part of the plant (28).

The general environment in an area affected by a toxic release (e.g., by a plume of gas or a chemical deposit) should be carefully examined for effects on animals, vegetation and artifacts. Illness and death in animals may be the first indication of a health hazard to man and this has been documented in the incidents at Minamata (cat dancing disease); Seveso (deaths of rabbits, chickens and birds due to dioxin); the deaths of birds, cats, dogs, and horses in arenas in Missouri led to the discovery of a widespread dioxin contamination of soil (29); in Japan the deaths of broiler chickens could have alerted public health officials to a hazard from the PCBs in the Yusho incident; in the mix-up between the cattle feed and the fire-retardent in Michigan sickness in cattle first alerted officials to a risk to human milk and dairy products from polybrominated biphenyls. The state of health of animals and plants is therefore an important guide which was not appreciated at Seveso; hence the anomaly of not evacuating people in the contaminated zone until two weeks after the accident even though plants and animals had begun to die within a few days. Damage to vegetation can also be useful in determining in retrospect the path of a plume of toxic gas, as at Bhopal (30). In contrast, the absence of any damage to vegetation around Lake Nyos within the extensive area where people and animals were killed was a very important clue which refuted the opinion that the skin lesions in the victims had been caused by an acidic gas or by heat (10). The state of artifacts such as plastics, newspaper, wooden furniture, clothing, etc., will provide useful information on the likely thermal or blast impact on man if these have been involved. After volcanic eruptions information on the carbonization of wood, softening of plastics, charring of newspaper, etc., assists in identifying the temperatures which have been achieved in areas of destruction. Little information is available on the best methods of detecting chemical residues in the environment after an industrial release. Some chemicals, such as dioxin or chlorinated hydrocarbon pesticides, are very resistant to environmental degradation but the value of emergency testing for residues of other chemicals is not proven. On the other hand, deposits of chemical dust on the ground in inhabited areas should be subjected to urgent analysis in order to determine whether a health hazard exists or not. A state of readiness in appropriate national laboratories should always exist so that tests can be performed at any time of the day or night regardless of the day of the week. This point failed to be appreciated at a fire in a warehouse containing 2000 tons of chemicals in a built-up area in Salford, England, in 1982, which resulted in hundreds of evacuated people being returned to their homes in a heavily contaminated area; fortunately the layer of dust proved to be of lower toxicity than it might have been, given the array of substances that could have been stored on-site (31). The investigation of the Toxic Oil Syndrome showed the inadequacy of containing samples of suspect edible oil when the epidemic was on the wane, by which time samples containing the chemical contaminant could already have been consumed or thrown away. When a toxic cause is suspected in an outbreak of illness, samples of dairy products (meat, milk, eggs), alcoholic beverages, drinking water (and fish, if a staple food), flour, and edible oils should be sought early on from affected households and stored for subsequent analysis, otherwise a bolus of chemical contamination could be missed. These five vehicles have been the most prominent in previous outbreaks involving food or drink (1).

7. Toxicological

All the above approaches are observational, or descriptive, and as such have certain scientific limitations. The opportunity to observe a repetition of disastrous incident to test a hypothesis generated by investigators after a first event is most unlikely to occur (though a similar outbreak to Yusho occurred in Taiwan in 1979). Thus, from the scientific viewpoint, the ability to reproduce the disease in animals using the suspect material may be indispensable in demonstrating a causal link. Conversely, the absence of a laboratory animal model and the failure to induce the disease by experimentation may leave many unconvinced as to the causal agent, particularly when the results may be used to impute blame in an industrial disaster. Various specimens of rape seed oil supposedly from affected households in the toxic oil syndrome were tested in animals, but without success, and so the causal agent in this outbreak remains unidentified. In vitro and in vivo laboratory testing is of great importance in the screening of chemicals for use in industry and extensive testing of chemical agents, as well as long-term epidemiological follow-up of the exposed, may therefore be an important part of the research effort for many years after a disaster has occurred.

EVALUATING THE EVIDENCE

The investigative team will collect information of variable quality and quantity, and an inadequate emergency response may make the drawing of firm conclusions on a causal link between a health effect and a putative agent impossible. In the place of strong evidence several different competing hypotheses may emerge to explain the event, and political or legal considerations may begin to overwhelm scientific objectivity. Reliance may have to be placed on almost entirely observational rather than experimental, toxicologicl evidence. How should the investigators proceed in these circumstances?

The dilemma posed by insufficient information was dramatically illustrated at the Lake Nyos disaster, though similar considerations apply to Bhopal and to the Toxic Oil Syndrome. The phenomenon at Lake Nyos had no precedent, except for a little-known incident at Lake Monoun in Cameroon where 39 people were killed in a gas release almost two years before (10). The controversy at Lake Nyos revolved around whether gas had been released from a volcanic eruption or a gas burst for the lake itself. Some of the local people did not agree with either of these hypotheses, and believed that the event had been causes by a military device (perhaps a neutron bomb) detonated by a foreign country. No doubt even more fanciful explanations were being put about as well. The failure of scientists to agree opened the door to the more dubious explanations, with the danger that agreement on the preventive measures needed to avoid a further loss of life from a repetition of the gas release would not be reached.

Scientists do not approach the world with an open mind which collects a mass of unprejudiced observations from which the underlying causes or explanations can be discovered (the "inductive" process). According to Briskman (32), who follows Karl Popper, empirical support can be found for almost any theory so long as we look for it. Thus we can say that "in the absence of any empirical means of eliminating either of (two theories) as false the fact that both can be shown to agree with many observed facts says

TABLE 1

EXAMPLES OF ACUTE CHEMICAL INCIDENTS

WATER

ADDITIVES:

Sodium hydroxide (USA, 1980)
Fluoride (USA, 1979)
Aluminum sulphate (UK, 1988)

CONTAMINANTS:
Chlordane (USA, 1876, 1980)
Phenol (UK, 1984)

FOOD AND DRINK

ADDITIVES:

Flour Niacin (USA, 1980, 1983)
Margarine Potassium bromate (S. Africa, 1968)
Beer Cobalt (Quebec, 1965)

CONTAMINANTS:

Alcoholic drink manufacture Lead
(moonshine), TOCP (ginger root)
Edible oil distribution Tri-ortho-cresyl phosphate (drums)
Food Crops Aldicarb (watermelons, cucumbers)
Flour production (home-made) Lead
(W.Bank, 1982)
Flour transportation Parathion (Sierra Leone, 1986)
Endrin (UK, 1956)
Methylene dianiline (UK, 1965)

TABLE 2

EXAMPLES OF CHRONIC DISORDERS REPORTED IN MAJOR CHEMICAL INCIDENTS

Carginogenic	Polychlorinated biphenyls (Japan)
Teratogenic	Organic mercury (Japan)
Immunological	Polybrominated biphenyls (Michigan)
Neurological	Tri-o-cresyl phosphate (eg USA, 1930)
Pulmonary	Methyl isocyanate (India)
Hepatic	Benzene Hexachloride (Turkey)
Dermatological	Toxic oil syndrome (Spain)

not a jot for the truth of either" (32). Instead, the scientific worth of a theory should not be gauged on the abundance of evidence in its favor but whether the theory is capable of being empirically refuted.

Scientific dispute may be good for the souls of researchers but it leaves the decision-makers frustrated and impotent. It therefore behooves the scientific investigators not merely to express honest disagreement but to put forward an agreed plan by which the competing theories can be eliminated through further information-gathering and a process of refutation using the multidisciplinary approach outlined above.

CONCLUSION

The purpose of this chapter was to propose that the successful management of a toxic disaster depends upon the urgent involvement of scientists from a select range of disciplines, none of which can necessarily provide sufficient information alone. The control of major toxic hazards in industry has already produced the necessary skills but apart from the laboratory and toxicological disciplines the others all need to be performed on, or close to, the scene of the disaster. The medical management of many previous major incidents can readily be faulted because of a failure to rapidly mobilize or coordinate the multidisciplinary team needed, thereby leaving unfillable gaps in evaluating the risk to populations or understanding how the disaster occurred (1). Public health officials need to be aware of the complexities of dealing with toxic releases compared with other types of disaster, and that the expertise required for managing such incidents may be beyond local or even national resources. Much more medical planning and coordination on an international as well as national level needs to go into toxic disaster preparedness in both developed and developing nations than has been apparent so far.

REFERENCES

1. Baxter, PJ, in press: Review of major chemical incidents and their medical management. Proc. Roy. Soc. Med.

2. Magos L, 1988: Thoughts on life with untested and adequately tested chemicals. Br. J. Ind. Med., 45: 721-726.

3. Royal Society of Medicine, 1976: Vinyl chloride. Meeting of the Section of Occupational Medicine. Proceeding of the Royal Society of Medicine, 69: 275-310.

4. Baxter PJ, Anthony PP, MacSween RNM, Schever PJ, 1977: Angiosarcoma of the liver in Great Britain, 1963-73. Br. Med. J., 2:913-974.

5. Baxter PJ, Anthony PP, MacSween RNM, Schever PJ, 1980: Angiosarcoma of the liver: incidence and aetiology in Great Britain. Br. J. Ind. Med., 37:213-221.

6. Fox AJ, Collier PF, 1977: Mortality experience of workers exposed to vinyl chloride monomer in the manufacture of polyvinyl chloride in Great Britain. Br. J. Ind. Med., 34:1-10.

7. Falk H, Baxter PJ, 1981: Hepatic angiosarcoma registries: implications for rare-tumor studies. Banbury Report 9: Quantification of Occupational Cancer, Coldspring Harbour Laboratory.

8. Buist AS, Bernstein RS (eds), 1986: Health effects of volcanoes: an approach to evaluating the health effects of an environmental hazard. Am. J. Public Health, 76 (suppl.): 1-90.

9. Merchant JA, 1986: Preparing for disaster. Am. J. Pub. Health, 76:233-235.

10. Baxter PJ, Kapila M, Mfonfu D, 1989: Lake Nyos disaster, Cameroon, 1986: the medical effects of large scale emission of carbon dioxide? Br. Med. J., 298: 1437-1441.

11. World Health Organization, 1984: Toxic Oil Syndrome. Copenhagen: WHO.

12. Tsubaki T, Irukayama K (eds), 1977: Minamata Disease. Elsevier Scientific Publishing Co, Amsterdam.

13. Amin-Zaki L, Majeed MA, Clarkson TW, Greenwood MR, 1978: Methyl mercury poisoning in Iraqi children: clinical observations over two years. Br. Med. J., 1:613.616.

14. Cripps DJ, Peters HA, Gocmen A, Dogramici I, 1984: Porphyria Turcica due to hexachlorobenzene: a 20-30 year follow-up study on 204 patients. Br. J. Dermatol., 111:413-422.

15. Senanayake N, Jeyaratnam J, 1981: Toxic polyneuropathy due to gingli oil contaminated with tri-cresyl phosphate affecting adolescent girls in Sri Lanka. Lancet, 1:88-89.

16. Doeglas HMG, Hermans EH, Huisman J, 1961: The Margarine Disease. Arch. Dermatol., 83-837-843.

17. Kuratsune M, Yoshimura T, Matsuzaka J, Yamaguchi A, 1971: Yusho, a poisoning caused by rice oil contaminated with polychlorinated biphenyls. HSMHA Health Reports, 86:1083-1091.

18. Hay A, 1982: The chemical scythe. New York: Plenum Press.

19. Kopelman H, Schever PJ, Williams R, 1966: The liver lesion of the Epping Jaundice. Quart. J. Med., 35: 553-564.

20. Eisele JW, O'Halloran RL, Reay DT, Lindholm GR, Lewman LV, Brady WJ, 1981: Deaths during the May 18, 1980, eruption of Mount St. Helens. New Eng. J. Med., 305:931-936.

21. Centers for Disease Control, 1988: Preliminary Report: 2,3,7,8,-tetra-chlorobenzo-p-dioxin. Exposure to humans - Seveso, Italy. MMWR, 37:733-736.

22. Halbert FL, Jackson TF, 1974: A toxic syndrome associated with the feeding of polybrominated biphenyl-contaminated protein concentrate to dairy cattle. J. Am. Vet. Med. Assoc., 165:437-439.

23. Brilliant LB, van Amburg G, Isbister J, et al, 1978: Breast milk monitoring to measure Michigan's contamination with polybrominated biphenyls. Lancet, 2:643-646.

24. Drotman DP, Baxter PJ, Liddle JA, Brokopp CD, Skinner MD, 1983: Contamination of the food chain by poly-chlorinated biphenyls from a broken transformer. Am. J. Pub. Health, 73:290-292.

25. Kreiss K, Zack MM, Kimbrough RD, Needham LL, Smrek AL, Jones BT, 1981: Cross-sectional study of a community with exceptional exposure to DDT. J. Am. Med. Assoc., 245:1926-1930.

26. Anonymous editorial, 1989: Asthma and the bean. Lancet, 2:538-540.

27. Ashley DL, Needham LL, 1986: Assessments of a scheme for prioritizing inorganic toxicants by using signs-and-symptoms analysis. Clin. Toxicol., 24:375-387.

28. Varma DR, 1989: Hydrogen cyanide and Bhopal. Lancet, 2:567-568.

29. Patterson DG, Hoffman RE, Needham LL, et al, 1986: 2,3,7,8-tetra-chlorodibenzo-p-dioxin levels in adipose tissue of exposed and control persons in Missouri. JAMA, 256:2683-2686.

30. Singh MP, Ghosh S, 1987: Bhopal gas tragedy: model simulation of the dispersion scenario. J. Hazard. Mat., 17:1-22.

31. Health & Safety Executive, 1983: The fire and explosions at B & R Hauliers, Salford, 25 September 1982. London: HMSO.

32. Briskman L, 1987: Doctors and witch doctors: which doctors are which? Parts 1 & 2. Br. Med. J., 295:1033-1036; 1108-1110.

THE AIRCRAFT DISASTER

John C. Duffy, M.D., FAPA, FAsMA

Assistant Surgeon General, U.S. Public Health Service
U.S.A.

INTRODUCTION

The number 25 was to have a somber significance for commercial aviation in the United States of America. It was on September 25, 1978, that what was at the time identified as the worst aviation disaster in U.S. history occurred, when two planes collided in the air over the city of San Diego. In that crash, PSA Flight 182, a Boeing 727 jetliner, and a Cessna single-engine plane collided while traveling in the same direction. Both planes plummeted immediately to the ground, killing a total of 144 persons. The death toll comprised all passengers aboard the two aircrafts and seven people who were either in homes or on the street at the point of impact. Of the 135 persons on board the PSA flight, 39 were employees of the company.

It was on another 25th day of the month (this time in May, 1979) when a wide-bodied DC-10 jetliner plummeted to earth moments after takeoff at O'Hare International Airport in Chicago, Illinois, killing all 270 persons aboard. This achieved the new title of the worst air disaster in the United States aviation history. American Flight 191, nonstop for Los Angeles, had just taken off from runway 32 right, headed northwest. Immediately after takeoff, the left engine separated from the aircraft. Then, from an altitude of approximately 200 feet, it nosed down, and burst into flame and smoke that could be seen up to eight miles away.

In both accidents, the effects were devastating. People were decapitated, cremated, blown to pieces and dismembered in horrifying ways. As an observer with the National Transportation and Safety Board, I was to participate in every phase of the events following the May 25, 1979, accident. My purpose was to identify the points of maximal emotional stress in such an experience and to suggest intervention strategies to mitigate the severe psychological impact.

BACKGROUND

Disaster studies have evolved from primarily descriptive field studies to the more recent efforts which are highly analytical and systematic. In 1976, Manning published a comprehensive bibliography, Disasters Technology(1), in which are listed several hundred references which focus on diverse areas of disaster research, including the sociological and psychological effects of disasters.

Health and Medical Aspects of Disaster Preparedness
Edited by J.C. Duffy
Plenum Press, New York, 1990

The findings from these studies suggest that subsequent to disasters, most individuals adapt, equilibrium is finally regained, or a reconstruction takes place in which a completely new equilibrium is established.(2) Thus, there appears to exist a process of reorganization in which trauma victims move from a place of chaos to one of order. Apparently, this process is a function of time and it is at a point on the adjustment continuum, where the traumatic experience becomes tolerable to the individual, letting a new equilibrium or reorganization take place, leaving the individual changed in some manner. Therefore, even though the effects of a trauma subside, there may be, as Moore and Associates(3) suggest, a long-term emotional residual of the traumatic event. Clinicians have generally recognized that rage, torture, and self-recrimination are hallmarks of frustrated grief and submerged mourning.(4)

Eight survivors of the worst aviation disaster in history (namely the Santa Cruz de Tenerife Island accident) were interviewed five months after it occurred. The survivors were still experiencing many of the symptoms of traumatic neurosis, as delineated by Fenichel.(5) Six other survivors were interviewed and findings indicated that one year after the disaster, survivors were in the reorganizational phase of adjustment. Responses of all subjects had changed significantly from responses given during the interviewing and testing seven months earlier. Those individuals who had suffered most, however, had not made as many adaptive changes, and were still exhibiting some of the post-traumatic neuroses.

Earlier studies of war neuroses provide evidence that there might be later arousal of trauma, even though pathology may not be present immediately following the extreme stress.(6,7) Other investigators have emphasized that even though shock may last only a few hours or, at most, days, no one can be certain that the remission of symptoms indicates entire recovery.(2) Still other investigators (8) further suggest that the majority of people who experience a disaster even indirectly (through identifying themselves with the victims or victim population) may also experience some degree of emotional upset in the period following the disaster. In other words, even those support personnel who assist the survivors at a disaster scene experience emotional symptomotology similar to that experienced by the actual victims of the disaster.

DISCUSSION

Crisis mental health intervention in a commercial aircraft accident can play a significant role in reducing the mental anguish and psychiatric consequences of such an accident. However, my own personal experience in the Chicago disaster reinforces my belief that there is an unwillingness to confront this issue. Rescuers were will prepared to mount an aggressive course of action in terms of collecting a group of specialists in Forensic Pathology to accomplish the rather difficult and complex task of body identification. On the other hand, they remained unaware of the <u>human</u> tragedy of such an event. Clearly, no airline company wishes to face the reality of one of its airplanes involved in an accident. Nevertheless, because of the increasing number of victims, airlines and airports must forthrightly address the issues involved, develop the necessary plans, provide the education of their personnel, and in general, respond in a more positive fashion towards a much more serious issue in the accident - that is, its emotional impact.

What do we know about individuals who experience such an extreme stress, "the disaster syndrome"? It has been described as a three-stage process which includes: (1) the "shock stage," (2) the suggestible stage," and (3) the "recovery stage."(9) In the shock stage, the victim is so dazed and stunned that he is likely to wander about aimlessly and is unable to help either himself or others; he may even become stuporous, disoriented or even amnesic concerning the traumatic event. During the suggestible stage, the victim passively accepts guidance, as his performance remains highly inefficient. He may even regress to infantile dependence on another. Finally, with the recovery stage, he gradually regains control. None the less, tension, apprehension, and nightmares may persist in the individual and he may appear to have a persistent need to tell the story of the incident repeatedly. Feelings of guilt, extreme agitation, nightmares and a sense of impending doom may persist. The latter symptoms manifest themselves as a state of free-floating anxiety and severe depression. However, it has been found that if supportive therapy is given immediately after the calamitous incident, the shock symptoms abate rapidly.

In an aircraft accident, the target population includes survivors, relatives, friends, air crew members, and rescue personnel. Reflecting both upon the ill-fated PSA Flight 182 of September 25, 1978, and the American Airlines Flight 191 of May 25, 1979, I should also like to suggest that the "victims" of the disaster were not only the passengers of the plane among whom there were no survivors. Rather, the psychological or secondary victims were those on the ground at the crash site, the emergency personnel, police, and the firemen, the emergency medical technicians who suddenly found themselves amid the debris tasked to pack up the tattered bits of human flesh.

Who then are the stress victims of an air disaster? Of course, if there are survivors, both passengers and crew members come to mind first. The families of the injured and the deceased also experience the emotional impact of the crash, including the relief workers, as already noted. Airport personnel and government airline administrators may also be prone to the effects of fatigue and stress, at a time when their decisions and leadership are crucial to the rescue effort.

What then are the emotional problems which must be faced? The typical emergency scenario can be divided into three chronological categories: pre-crash, crash and crash site (short-range problems), and post-crash (long-range problems). Once the crew members learn of the inevitability of the crash, they are faced with the problem of how to warn the passengers of the imminent danger. Research shows that the more time people have to absorb such news and prepare for the eventuality, the better they are able to cope with the situation.

At the crash site, the trauma of the situation can produce a host of reactions. Victims may exhibit symptoms of apathy, hysteria, non-comprehension, disorientation, regression, and extreme dependency. The friends of the victim may experience anxiety, anger, and grief. Rescue workers and care-givers are prone to the "burnout" syndrome which is characterized by exhaustion, irritability, and fatigue. This seriously hampers their critical judgment and capability. Although these symptoms may appear obvious to others, those experiencing the "burnout" syndrome fail to recognize it in themselves. Long-range problems are defined as those which manifest themselves after the emergency stage of the crash is over. Those affected by the accident may exhibit such chronic problems as withdrawal from employment, family life, psychosomatic ailments, or habitual anxiety. Survivors often experience a sense of guilt. They are plagued by two questions, "Why did I not do more to save those who perished?" and "Why did I survive and others did not?" Victims may experience greater episodes of depression and anxiety, on or about the anniversary of the disaster. This phenomenon has been appropriately labeled the "anniversary syndrome," and may occur without the conscious understanding of the victim.

TRAINING

How do you identify and train mental health workers for air disaster relief assignments? Who coordinates and has jurisdiction over such efforts? Due to the interstate and international characteristics of air travel, these problems do not yield any easy solution.

Because victims are often dispersed to various care facilities and then return as quickly as possible to their homes, there is the imposed difficulty of providing both acute care at the crash site, as well as long-term follow-up treatment and assessment. Who is responsible for the provision of crisis intervention? The airlines, the government, the mental health centers are all possibilities. Additional problems to be faced include how are families of the deceased informed of their loss with the least amount of traumatic impact. How is the grim task of identification of remains handled? How is the situation handled at the crash site when the need for information about the disposition of the flight often spawns many, sometimes inflammatory, rumors?

Every one of these questions surfaced without answers during my involvement with the Flight 191 accident. It is clear that these compelling questions, having already been proposed in a conference in Hilton Head in 1978, have yet to be addressed by the airline industry. In spite of all of the problems, my experience in Chicago suggests that there are steps that can be taken to improve the situation. Methods already exist where effective mental health crisis intervention has been provided in the aftermath of the natural disaster. Further, the airlines already have a disaster plan that focuses on the medical aspects of delivering aid to crash victims and that contains solutions for some of the logistical issues already raised. These plans can be modified to include crisis mental health services. Some airline companies have now developed a "psychological" plan along with their crash response scenario.

In such a brief presentation, it would not be possible to deal in any great detail regarding the specifics of training in crisis mental health intervention which could be provided to airline personnel and others. But techniques are available for developing the necessary skills; among them are included instruction through lectures, the use of training manuals, role-playing and videotape practice sessions, desensitizing for feelings of distress of repugnance when exposed to death or injury, and trainee visits to hospitals, mortuaries, and morgues in an effort to condition through exposure to the injured and dead.

RECOMMENDATIONS

As already mentioned, the emotional sequel of an aircraft disaster is both short-term and long-term in nature. Inclusion of mental health professionals in the response group to an accident would be of considerable help in dealing with the short-term mental health aspects of the crisis. Obviously, a handful of health professionals cannot do that alone; therefore, it would be important that all airport personnel receive training in how to handle people traumatized by an air disaster. This training should not only be cognitive and instructive, but also experimental, through use of encounter techniques, videotape interviews of victims and bereaved families, and other techniques of rehearsal. They would also prepare the crew for handling the crisis during the pre-crash phase. The mental health services provided only during the immediate post-crash are not sufficient and indeed emotional breakdown can occur long after the crash has been cleared and the physical injuries have been attended to. Victims should be encouraged to seek out professional mental health services in their community, either through their physicians or the federally-funded community mental health centers.

SUMMARY

We can no longer ignore the mass tragedy of a wide bodied aircraft accident. We are dealing potentially in the thousands, in terms of victims and affected individuals. We can ill afford to ignore this most critical issue, or worse, to respond to it with defensiveness or a naive interpretation of the problem. Consequently, I would like to make the following recommendation: establishment of an information clearing house on the psychological aspects of aircraft disasters. It is essential to collect hard data on the emotional aspects of aircraft disasters so that the industry cannot easily dismiss the goals of providing crisis mental health intervention.

Certainly, insurance companies can provide an additional impetus to the adoption of mental health service on the part of the airlines. Having been exposed to neurosis claims on the part of natural disaster victims, they can sensitize the airlines to the likelihood of similar claims against air carriers winning favorable decisions from the courts. Underwriters can help in other ways as well by altering rate structures, by providing financial incentives, and by assisting in the preparation of disaster relief protocols with a mental health component.

References

1. Manning, Diana Helen: *Disaster Technology: an annotated bibliography*. New York: Pergamon Press, 1976.

2. Wilson, Robert N. "Disaster and Mental Health," *In Man and Society in Disaster*, edited by G.W. Baker and D.S. Chapman. New York: Basic Books, 1962.

3. Moore, H.E. *Tornadoes Over Texas: A study of Waco and San Angelo in Disaster*. Austin, Texas: University of Texas Press, 1958.

4. Figley, C.R. Symptoms of delayed combat stress among a college sample of Vietnam veterans. *Military Medicine* 143 (2): 107-110, Feb. 1978.

5. Fenichel, O. Concept of trauma in contemporary psychoanalytical theory. *International Journal of Psycho-Analysis* 26: 33-44, 1945.

6. Grinker, R., Spiegel, J.P. *Men Under Stress*. Philadelphia, Blakiston, 1945.

7. Segal, J.; Hunter, E.J.; Segal, Z. Universal consequences of captivity: stress reactions among divergent populations of prisoners of war and their families. *International Social Science Journal* 28 (3): 593-609, 1976.

8. Fritz, C.E., Williams, H.B. The human being in disasters: A research perspective. *Ann. Amer. Acad. Pol. and Soc. Sci.* 309: 42-51, 1957.

9. Goldenson, Robert M. *The Encyclopedia of Human Behavior*. vol. 1. New York, Doubleday, 1970. pp. 211-212.

INDEX